My Father's Heart

Also by Steve McKee

The Call of the Game

Coach: America's coaches of all kinds of sports, from the peewees to the pros, talk about the game, the players, building the team, the sacrifices, the pressure, winning and losing, their worst moments and their finest

My

FATHER'S
HEART

A Son's Journey

Steve McKee

Da Capo
LIFE
LONG

A MEMBER OF THE PERSEUS BOOKS GROUP

Brigadoon excerpt courtesy of The Alan Jay Lerner Testamentary Trust. *Brigadoon* was copyrighted in 1947 by Alan Jay Lerner and Frederick Loewe, copyright renewed.

In a few instances names and identifying characteristics of people in this book have been changed.

Portions of this book previously appeared in altered form in the *Wall Street Journal* and WSJ.com; *Alaskafest*, an early Alaska Airlines in-flight magazine; and *Alaska Today*, a journalism department publication of the University of Alaska–Fairbanks.

Designed by Timm Bryson
Set in 11 point New Caledonia by the Perseus Books Group

Library of Congress Cataloging-in-Publication Data
McKee, Steve.
My father's heart : a son's journey / Steve McKee. -- 1st Da Capo Press ed.
p. cm.
ISBN-13: 978-0-7382-1097-1 (alk. paper)
ISBN-10: 0-7382-1097-8 (alk. paper)
1. McKee, Steve--Health. 2. McKee, John, 1919-1969--Death. 3. Myocardial infarction--Patients--United States--Biography. 4. Cardiovascular system--Diseases--Patients--United States--Biography. 5. Coaches (Athletics)--United States--Biography. 6. Fathers and sons--United States--Biography. I. Title.
RC685.I6M42 2008
362.196'12370092--dc22
[B]
2007035613

Published by Da Capo Press
A Member of the Perseus Books Group
www.dacapopress.com

Da Capo Press books are available at special discounts for bulk purchases in the United States by corporations, institutions, and other organizations. For more information, please contact the Special Markets Department at the Perseus Books Group, 2300 Chestnut Street, Suite 200, Philadelphia, PA 19103, or call (800) 255-1514, or e-mail special.markets@perseusbooks.com.

1 2 3 4 5 6 7 8 9

To my sister, Kathy,
who lived this same story differently

In memory of
Alice McKee Murphy
November 21, 1923–January 15, 2007

and

Helen O'Neil McKee
December 24, 1920–October 13, 2007

PROLOGUE

The first call went to my sister, living in Florida.

It's happening. It's really happening.

This book project was still in its earliest stages, but it had reached that point where everyone involved—author, agent, editor—has by consensus agreed that the deal has been done. Nothing has been signed yet, however, so of course it hasn't. But at the same time it has, just about, meaning the author, fairly bursting with news and desperate to tell people, begins . . . to tell people. So I called my sister, Kathy.

It's all done but the signing, Kath. I know it ain't over till it's over . . . but it's over. It's going to happen, this book I have been writing all my life. . . .

I *have* been writing this book all my life, or at least for most of it. In the fall of 1973, twenty years old, I took a writing course during my senior year at Allentown College of St. Francis de Sales in Pennsylvania. For the opening assignment there was no other moment to consider than the events of Tuesday, September 30, 1969, rendered in barely fictionalized form.

Twenty-eight years after that September night, now a copy editor at the *Wall Street Journal*, some of what I'd written in college, remade now as wholly true, appeared nearly verbatim in an essay I wrote for one of the paper's special health sections. Seven years after that, in another *Journal Report*, I brought the story full circle and up to date. And twice while writing for WSJ.com, the online *Journal*, I culled specific moments from those events of long ago, fleshing them out into their own remembrances.

I know, Kath, I know—be careful what you wish for—but it's happening.

Kathy let a short silence hang between us on the phone.

"I hope," she finally said, "I hope that when you're done with this that you'll like Dad more and think better of him." She said it without malice, without judgment. Still, her comment stung. Like Dad more? Think better of him? I already do. Of course I do. He's . . . Dad.

"And I hope," she said, "I hope you can forgive him for dying when he did, and the way he did."

Today, nearly 80 million adults in this country have cardiovascular disease in one form or another (or possibly in combination). That's one out of every three Americans. Cardiovascular disease—high blood pressure, coronary heart disease, stroke, etc.—is the underlying cause of one of every three deaths in the United States each year. Every day, nearly 2,400 Americans die of cardiovascular disease's major heart breakers. That's one death every thirty-six seconds. If we could wave a magic wand and eliminate this scourge, we could all expect to live nearly seven years longer. If only.

Approximately 16 million people in the United States have coronary heart disease. In the next 12 months, approximately 700,000 Americans will experience a myocardial infarction; a heart attack. Another 500,000 will experience their second myocardial infarction, or perhaps their third or fourth. In addition there will likely be a third group of perhaps 175,000 who will experience a myocardial infarction, but not know they did. And in the next year, 325,000 people will die from what is termed "out-of-hospital" or "emergency room" sudden cardiac arrest —the classic heart attack of popular lore, just like Dad's on September 30, 1969. It was just the two of us at home that night. He was fifty; I was sixteen.

"Diseases of the heart," as termed by government nomenclature, have been the leading cause of death in the United States since 1910. Pneumonia and influenza had a three-year-run at number one in 1918, 1919, and 1920, but heart disease reclaimed the top spot in 1921, and it has not been headed since. Cardiovascular disease attacks across all lines: gender, race, and ethnicity. Paint a map of the United States with the color red to indicate where the death rate by cardiovascular disease is highest, and the eastern half would be a far darker crimson than the barely pink western half. In that eastern portion the southern quadrant would be such a deep red as to be a death-like purple. Within this broad picture there are insidious brush strokes. African-American men, for instance, are much more likely than white men and far more likely than Hispanic men to die of heart disease. Among women, African Americans again have the highest heart-disease mortality rate.

And cardiovascular disease is relentless. A forty-year-old man who today is free of the disease has a 2-in-3 chance of having it by age seventy; for women the chance is about 1-in-2. Cardio-vascular disease annually costs this country more than $400 billion in health-care expenditures and lost productivity. To break some figures out: hospital care, $133 billion; doctor and clinic fees, more than $40 billion; prescription drugs, nearly $50 billion.

Eventually, however, the numbers, the stats, the dollars—they stop the heart itself. They overwhelm the senses; they boggle the mind. They mean everything; they mean nothing. Ultimately, they lose their power. Heart disease, because it is everywhere, sometimes appears to be nowhere. "He died of a heart attack," has about it an almost natural ring. It shouldn't.

Here's a new equation. All the people who in the next twelve months will succumb to cardiovascular disease, heart disease, and heart attacks were each some combination (surely multifaceted) of husband or wife, son or daughter, brother or sister, mother or father, grandma or grandpa. Each was a friend or lover, coworker or acquaintance, boss or valued lieu-tenant, fishing partner or fellow churchgoer, next-door neigh-bor or the after-school carpool driver for Thursday's swim club. Each was a Little League coach or den mother, teacher or doctor, the friendliest checkout clerk at the drugstore or the guy who spotted you at the gym during the bench press. By this calculation, first the lives and then the deaths of every one of these people will affect millions, millions, *millions* of others.

I know. It happened to me. It is the story I've been writing all my life. The father leaves; the son remains. If it is an extraordinary tale, it is so only in the fact that it is ordinary. Should there be power here, that's where I'll find it. My father died on a Tuesday. I returned to my high school, to my senior year, the next Tuesday, October 7, 1969. I will start there, at school, and journey across those eight days to that final night.

My father died before I knew him. I hope, through this, to understand him now. He also died before he knew me. There is no changing that, but if I can discover him, what might I learn of myself? I hope these pages enlighten on the subject of heart disease—I most surely do—but this isn't intended as a self-help tome. I want this to provide information for people affected by this number-one killer, but I am not writing a how-to book. I am no expert, and I won't pretend to be one.

I am here simply to finish the story I have been writing all my life. Finally. Of one dad, one son, one family. Kathy had it almost correct. I hope when I have completed this that I will love my father more. But I hope it is he who can forgive me for not forgiving him.

TUESDAY, OCTOBER 7

FORJAN. THE APTLY NAMED JIM FORJAN. BECAUSE OVER THE FINAL four decades of the twentieth century his personality forged the very character of York Catholic High School, hammering it into tempered steel.

Relentless, unyielding, implacable. That was Jim Forjan. Blunt, brusque, brisk. Steadfast, resolute, principled. Tough, fair, honest. Eccentric, predictable, impulsive. Terrifying. That was Forjan, too.

And he was staring right at me.

He came to York Catholic in the fall of 1959 as the boys' varsity basketball coach. During his eleven years on the bench his teams were ferociously disciplined, every ounce of their talent squeezed out. He always dominated the local county public schools; the real competition was in the Central Penn Catholic League. Heartbreakers on the road against Our Lady of Lourdes up in Shamokin or in Harrisburg against Bishop McDevitt usually proved his undoing for the league title. But, as a smaller school, his York Catholic Fighting Irish then proceeded to the

1

State Class B tournament, where, it always seemed, the Scranton Cathedral Golden Lancers ended his season in the Eastern Regional. These games were at a "neutral" site—three hours away at the Scranton C.Y.O. court, where Cathedral played four or five games a year. We in York never understood the selection process.

On the sidelines he was a mess, a nervous wreck, a comical collection of elbows and knees, edges and points, everything looking for a place to sit down. He was all jutting jaw and crewcut, his apparent inability to control himself in full contrast to his green-and-gold team on the court.

And there he stood, rail thin, framed in the doorway of the study hall, glowering. And could he glower.

He was a history teacher, too, but truth be told, a lousy one. Pregame he was too nervous to teach; postgame he was either too devastated or too elated to concentrate. Not to worry, though. He was the boys' basketball coach—back then, the time-honored, not-so-whispered exemption—the mantle granting unassailable status. Then, before my junior year, in 1968, word got out that Coach Forjan had been named school disciplinarian. It proved a move of counterintuitive brilliance, a page from the playbook of Red Auerbach himself, the legendary coach of the legendary Boston Celtics of the 1950s and 1960s—and, perhaps not coincidentally, one of Forjan's idols. When Auerbach stepped down as coach, two years before, he had caught everyone off guard one last time by naming his talented, proud, enigmatic center, Bill Russell, to succeed him. On the Celtics, who better to control Russell than Russell? At York Catholic, who better to control Forjan than Forjan?

From the moment he moved into his new office next to the study hall, this Ichabod Crane of a basketball coach merely owned the school.

I knew he was staring at me because I was the only person in the room, by myself amid rows of desks. York Catholic was switching to flexible scheduling next year and had been experimenting this year to get ahead of the quirks. I was a quirk, an unaccounted-for square peg wandering the round hole of seventh period, stuck here in study hall as a result.

I had seen this Forjan stare many times before (though never so razored in on me), once right in this very place. In the spring of the previous year, our junior class had gathered here to protest the results of the recent primary election for school president. We caucused before homeroom, the word passed from locker to locker. We weren't going to class until—until!— the results were thrown out. Then, suddenly, there stood Forjan in the doorframe, staring. White shirt, laughably skinny tie, arms akimbo, steam rising. Our conclave went dead quiet. The study hall would empty now, he said. Period. The room cleared; the election proceeded. You did not want Forjan staring at you.

"Steve," he said now, his voice brusque and impatient.

"Coach?" Everyone called him Coach.

"Get in my office."

I ran through the list of possible infractions. But there were none. How could there be? Today was Tuesday, and I hadn't been in school since last Tuesday. Still, there had to be something. I had no choice but to get in his office.

And so it began. For the rest of my senior year, I lived for seventh-period study hall. No matter what else was going on, I knew that seventh period was waiting for me at the end of the day, where I would be in the presence of the man. It stuns me to realize today that he was only thirty-three years old. Sometimes we would talk. Sometimes we wouldn't. Sometimes he would talk and I would listen. Often we walked the halls together: showing the colors, he called it. Kids started asking me about it. "What's the deal with you and Forjan . . . walking the halls . . . seventh period?" I didn't answer. I had no answer. Coach told me to walk, so I walked. They would have, too. But I was thrilled they noticed.

That first day I squeezed myself into his tiny office and sat in the chair on the opposite side of the big wooden desk that filled the room. Well, here it was, I figured. I expected the question. *Tell me about it, what happened?* Since last Tuesday I'd been asked that by everyone. But Coach surprised me, and not for the last time. He didn't say a word. Not one. He just sat there, ignoring me, tending to the papers on his desk. I was Scrooge awaiting the second of the three Spirits—"being prepared for almost anything, he was not by any means prepared for nothing." Which is what I got from Coach until what seemed like the following Tuesday.

Then finally came, "How you doin'?" in that I-could-care tone of his. He didn't even look up.

"I'm okay, Coach," I said.

"No you're not," he said, swatting my words away as if he were Russell himself blocking a shot. "No you're not," he said again. "Your father just died."

True, although not "just." This was Tuesday. Dad had died last Tuesday. Fifty years, eight months, nine days old. A heart attack had slammed him off the back of the couch while we were watching television. He had been to the doctor's only days before—no reason, just a checkup—and been declared fine.

It had been just the two of us at home that night. Mom was playing cards at a friend's house, and my sister, Kathy, was up in Buffalo, New York, where she had gone to school. Our phone was out, so I ran to get Mom after a policeman—by pure, dumb luck—had cruised past. This past weekend, Mom and Kathy and I took Dad to Buffalo, his and Mom's home-town, to bury him.

Now I had returned to York Catholic, a senior in the Class of 1970 and glad to be back, not that it wasn't all completely weird. My current events had bestowed upon me a strange, unreal status. I was at the center of attention, though no one knew how to approach me, or what to say if they did. If only for today, I was part of the energy source around which the rest of the school revolved. That wasn't my usual position in the York Catholic solar system. Normally I orbited comfort-ably out around the third or fourth ring—close enough to feel the glow but not far enough to know the chill. Only once be-fore had gravitational forces pulled me so close to the York Catholic sun: the previous year, when I was the comedy side-kick in the school musical. Now here I was again, if for all the wrong reasons. It felt good anyway. The price was steep, but I hadn't asked to pay it.

Coach leaned closer to me across the desk, folding long, bony fingers one into the other. With his heavy, horn-rimmed glasses and his prominent, pointy nose, he was a hawk inspect-ing his prey.

"Your father just died and you'll never get over it," he said, attacking. He leaned back. His declaration—blunt and pointed, breathtakingly honest—somehow took the tension out of the air, out of the past week, and I was grateful for it. He didn't say anything for a while, letting it all settle. I for sure didn't say word one, content to remain forever here in the presence of the truth. How *do* you get over this? When Coach finally did speak, his voice was a kindly whisper, or at least nearly. "But you will get used to it," he said. Then he sprang forward, reached for a hall pass, and scribbled on it. "Now get outta here," he said, back to brusque, enough revealed for one day. There would be a seventh period tomorrow. "Take this to Sister Magdalen."

━━━━━

About two years before the heart attack that killed him, I had told Dad in so many words that if he didn't clean up his act, he'd be dead in five years. Quit the smoking, get some exercise, stop nailing himself to the cross of his job. We were sitting at the kitchen table, he and Mom and I. Kathy was away at school. Dad had already had one heart attack, in 1963, when he was forty-four. It had been such an obvious warning shot across the bow. How could he not have heard it, when I so clearly had? He looked straight at me and said, "You're right." I wanted to reach across the table, grab him by the collar of the white dress shirt he always wore to work, and shake him. All these years later, I still do.

Shake him for proving me right with years to spare. Shake him for the cigarette cough Kathy and I woke up to every morning of our lives. For missing my high school and college graduations, my wedding in 1978. For not being here for me and my wife, Noreen, to share with him the baby, Patrick, that we adopted in 1990. And for Mom, the former Helen Theresa O'Neil of Seneca Parkside, for being his widow for thirty-seven years, fifteen years longer than she was his wife.

The truth? I think Dad gave up. I do. His father, my grand-father, Jack McKee, died on July 6, 1941, of a "Probable Coronary Occlusion," according to the death certificate. *Probable* is wholly unnecessary here; we are talking McKee family history, after all. For Jack, and for my Dad, it came all of a sudden, out of the blue. Maybe Dad needed a Forjan to wag a finger at him. Maybe Dad never got used to it.

Jack McKee was fifty-three when he died, and Dad was twenty-two at the time. Mom says that Dad "adored his father." As he wrote home to his mother during World War II: "I'm glad you see a resemblance between myself and dad. I'm trying, you see, to be a good man." Jack McKee was a plasterer by trade, a staunch union man—Local #9 out of North Tonawanda. Despite his profession (though in a way because of it), he had beautiful, soft hands. The plaster dried them out terribly, so he took meticulous care. Every night, home from work and before reading the *Buffalo Evening News* in his rocking chair, he would sit at the kitchen table with a bottle of olive oil, kneading it into his hands and fingers. He belonged to the Buffalo Racing Pigeon Concourse, and he followed the horses, though not as a betting man. He also enjoyed the fights on the radio. What Irishman didn't? Jimmy Slattery from the Old First Ward won the New York State version of a world light-heavyweight title in 1927 and three years later won it again, barely holding off another Buffalo boy, Lou Scozza, in a fifteen rounder right there at the Buffalo Broadway Auditorium.

My grandfather's heart attack happened on the way back from a day at Sunset Bay, one of many Lake Erie vacation spots southeast of Buffalo. Jack was driving. Next to him was my grandmother. We grandkids would know her as "Nana." Jack always called her "Babe." Without warning he pulled his blue Plymouth to the side of the road. "Biddy," he said, "how about if you drive?"

"Biddy" was Mary Jane, his eighteen-year-old daughter. As with "Babe" for his wife, only Jack could call Mary Jane "Biddy." They were his nicknames. A thrilled Mary Jane—she had only recently gotten her license—took the keys and slipped behind the wheel. Jack, meanwhile, got in the back next to his other daughter, seventeen-year-old "Skipper." Her real name was Alice Elizabeth.

"Jack!" That was Nana talking—screaming, really—as she turned around to look at her husband. It is impossible to know what prompted her to say it, what she'd heard, what she knew in that instant. It all happened too quickly. Mary Jane hadn't even put the key in the ignition, and my Aunt Alice, next to her father, says she remembers hearing no sound. Maybe Nana knew something was amiss as soon as Jack pulled over and asked Mary Jane to drive. Jack always drove. Maybe after a quarter-century of marriage she just knew.

In the time it took her to turn around and scream, Jack's head had been thrown against the seat and held there. One time only his head went back, and that's how he stayed, un-moving. He had been to the doctor's only days before—no reason, just a checkup—and had been declared fine.

Alice was dispatched to find a phone to call John, her older brother, my father. They had all said goodbye only about an hour earlier in front of the Sunset Bay cottage that Dad and some of his buddies from the neighborhood had rented for the summer—eight guys, $13 each for the season. Alice, the kid sister, loved having a big brother if only because it meant there were always boys at the house on Rodney Avenue or, like now, down at the lake. This time, though, there were older girls there, too, John's age or thereabouts, from South Buffalo. They had rented a cottage a street or two away—with two live-in chaperones, of course.

So there had been many people to say goodbye to, some of whom the McKees had just said hello to for the first time. That included a twenty-year-old Helen O'Neil—Mom—from South Buffalo in the city's longtime Irish belly. Indeed, it had likely been Nana's desire to meet this girl whom her son had been going on about for three years now—"Mom," he'd been telling her, "she laughs at my jokes!"—that had brought the McKees down to Sunset Bay in the first place, after an early Sunday Mass at Blessed Trinity Church. Nana having now taken her measure, the McKees had then headed home. Dad, meanwhile, rode back with some of the guys from the lake.

By the time Alice got to a phone, hours had passed since that parting. Dad was already at the house on Rodney Avenue, a nondescript street hard by a quarry on Buffalo's East

Side. He was already in bed, up in the third-floor attic that as a kid he had shared with his older brother, Tom. Weekends at the lake were surely filled with lots of Utica Club beer and plenty of laughs but not much sleep. Monday morning and another day at Trico Products, where he worked in the traffic department, would dawn soon enough. When Alice rang the phone on the parlor floor—Parkside 5739—it went unanswered. Eventually she got ahold of Walter Doersam from across the street. He climbed the back stairs to the attic. Together the two drove back, looking for Jack's Plymouth. They found it, near Southwestern Boulevard and Camp Road in Hamburg. There was a lumpy white sheet spread out on the ground next to the car.

It was a solemn ride to Rodney Avenue that night. In five months plus a day Pearl Harbor would be attacked. For everyone in America the old world would be gone. The McKees in the blue Plymouth merely got a head start on the great upheaval. With Jack gone, so was "Biddy" and so was "Skipper." Only he could call them that. When they had been little and Nana would be off with her lady friends for a Saturday afternoon's shopping, Jack would often scrub the kitchen floor. He would sit his two girls on the kitchen table and give each a glass of water. When he needed to raise more suds in a particular spot, he would point to it, and Biddy and Skipper would take a drink, aim, and spit. Now all that gone.

Gone too was my father's nickname. Jack McKee called his second son "Steve." And, of course, only he could. I never learned where "Steve" had come from; I don't think Dad knew, either. But Steve it was; first for Dad as a nickname, then for me as a real name.

Dad rarely talked about his father, and he never told me anything about the day he died. Once Dad had got knocked on his back by that first heart attack in 1963, I think he never quite got up again. Born on January 21, 1919, he had grown up through the Depression, been a young man in World War II, and had been a married man with a family in the postwar boom. He'd worshiped in the church of the American Dream, a true believer in the up-by-your-bootstraps gospel. And he reaped what he sowed, in an unassuming, middle-class sort of way, fine by him. I think he came to see a price to be paid for all that, and so be it.

For the six-plus years between Dad's two heart attacks, we McKees lived in a surreal sort of suspended animation, treading carefully, wondering if—when?—the other shoe would drop, another coronary artery clog. He was forty-four when he had his first attack on February 2; mom was forty-two. My sister, Kathy, was in eighth grade; I was in fifth. Dad spent at least a month in York Hospital, most of the time flat on his back, for weeks not permitted even to lift his arms above his head. He spent six more weeks at home before going back to work as a traffic-management executive at Cole Steel Equipment, the office-furniture company that he had worked for in York since 1954. "The boss of the warehouse," as Kathy and I liked to say.

Dad back to work! Yes, that was the ticket, the "normal" to which we all aspired. And that's what we got, with a vengeance.

Dad loved what he did for a living. But he hated his job. The stress, the boss—one was the other, and he handled neither well. It all conspired to kill him; never will I think otherwise.

Returning Dad to work meant that Dad returned to cigarettes. Couldn't we see that coming? He started up again within months after getting back to his office on the second floor, with the wall of windows looking down on his warehouse of responsibility. It was during that period, between his attacks, when I first started running. It would be poetic to write that I was a sixteen-year-old exorcizing my father's demons by exercising my own, but it wouldn't be true. (Later it would be, but not right out of the blocks.) No, I started running in the fall of my junior year at York Catholic because I was determined to become the country's next great African-American sprinter.

I remain almost serious about that now. I was, then, for sure.

The 1968 Summer Olympics in Mexico City were held that October. I devoured every minute of ABC's nearly forty-four hours of coverage, thrilling to Jim McKay's "Live from Mexico City!" It seemed so magical, so impossible, to be watching it in our TV room on Stanford Drive in Haines Acres in the east end of York, Pennsylvania, barely north of Maryland—yet it was taking place in Mexico City, in Estadio Olympico.

Being the middle-class suburban white boy I most surely was, I should have wanted to become the next great backward-flopping high jumper (Dick Fosbury), pretty-boy pole vaulter (Bob Seagren), world's greatest athlete (Bill Toomey), or even ancient four-time gold-medal discus thrower (thirty-two-year-old Al Oerter). I followed all of them, too, but it was the U.S. male sprinters who held me in their sway.

Jim Hines and Charlie Greene went gold and bronze at 100 meters. Tommie Smith and John Carlos were first and third in the 200. Lee Evans, Larry James, and Ron Freeman swept the 400, with Lee Evans's world record good for nearly twenty years. There were also Willie Davenport and Erv Hall going one-two in the 110-hurdles. I lapped it up, all of it. And then Mel Pender, Ronnie Ray Smith, and Vince Matthews joined in to help win additional gold in the four-by-one-hundred and four-by-four-hundred relays. Together, these dozen African-American men and their eleven total medals constitute arguably the greatest U.S. male sprint team ever assembled.

My devotion to the Olympics was cemented. I spent every Saturday, it seemed, at the Martin Memorial Library devouring the Olympics section. In the spring of my senior year I traveled to Italy with the Latin club and Sister Magdalen. The Sistine Chapel, the Trevi Fountain—yeah, they were great. But I wanted to see the 1960 Olympic Stadium. On our last day, Sister Magdalen helped me find it. When we got there we walked completely around, but the place was locked up tight. "I'm going to go for a walk now, Steve," Sister Magdalen said. She shook a finger at me. "Don't you dare sneak in." With that she turned and disappeared around a corner. I sneaked in, took off my shoes and socks, and ran barefoot on the same track where America's Dave Sime had been edged by Germany's Armin Hary in the 100-meter dash.

Of course, at the 1968 Mexico Games all that accomplishment by those U.S. sprinters was lost forever, turned into something else, once Tommie Smith and John Carlos raised black-gloved fists on the victory stand after their 200-meter performance. It had been a terrific race. Smith and Carlos were members of Coach Bud Winter's famed "Speed City" crew out in San Jose, California, and both had figured prominently in the yearlong speculation that America's black athletes would boycott the Games—Smith especially, in solidarity with the Olympic Project for Human Rights.

Yet now here they were in Mexico City, running, and simply dazzling, with Jim McKay calling the race. Smith pushed off tentatively, nursing a pulled groin, unsure he could run at all. . . . *Carlos, as usual, has burst out of the blocks. . . .* Huge and powerful, he swept to a nearly two-meter lead before even hitting the straight. Then came the lithe and elegant Smith, in a sudden, startling burst. *Right now it's Carlos and Smith.* Then it was just Smith. . . . *Here comes Tommie . . .* taking command with 60 meters left. *Smith has done it, with his hands in the air!* His final six strides he ran with his arms overhead in thrilling jubilation, a smile of absolute and pure joy breaking open his goatee. Carlos, stunned, stumbled to third place behind Australia's Peter Norman. All of it was wonderful stuff.

And all of it was mere prologue. The image to come on the medals platform is now iconic. Black gloves on Smith's right and Carlos's left hands, their arms extended. Bowed heads. Black socks on shoeless feet. A lone black track shoe on each pedestal. Smith in black scarf; Carlos in African beads. Second-place Norman wearing an Olympic Project button in support. I look at that picture now and try to remember what I was thinking then. If it rocked my suburban world I can't conjure it. Or perhaps with the advantage of all this hindsight I know better than to say so.

I was fifteen years old, for the one time in my life. And it had already been a tumultuous year. Everything was new to me; perhaps this was just more of the same. In January, North Korea boarded the USS *Pueblo*. In February, the Tet Offensive on television brought the look of defeat to Vietnam. In March, President Johnson declared that he would not run again. In April, Martin Luther King, Jr., was gunned down on a balcony in Memphis. In May, student riots in Paris nearly toppled President de Gaulle. In June, Bobby Kennedy was killed in a hotel kitchen in Los Angeles. In July, Pope Paul VI promulgated *Humanae Vitae*. In August, Chicago police battled antiwar protestors at the Democratic National Convention, and the Soviet Union marched into Czechoslovakia. In September, in Mexico City, the confrontation between students and riot police continued; eventually, hundreds would be killed after the *granaderos* opened fire. Later in October, Jackie Kennedy married Aristotle Onassis. And in November, a mean-spirited presidential campaign would grind to an end with Richard Nixon beating Hubert Humphrey in something of a dead heat, with the third-party candidate, George Wallace, taking nearly 14 percent of the vote. Not until December would there be good news, something to cheer for, to cheer us. The North Koreans released the *Pueblo* crew, and late night on December 24, the astronauts of *Apollo 8* circled the moon, read from Genesis, and gave us all a first look at a lonely Earth, lost in space.

Was I aware of this? Any of it? A fair question, and the answer is no. I was a kid, well sheltered in my suburbia. But the answer is also yes, because how could I not have been? I woke up every morning to the latest Vietnam body count. Bobby Kennedy was killed late at night in California; I heard that on the morning radio, too, and reported it to Mom and Dad. On Monday, October 21, all anyone in the halls of York Catholic was talking about before homeroom was the Kennedy-Onassis marriage. *How could she?* This was not idle gossip. The importance of the JFK presidency to this outpost of Catholics in south-central Pennsylvania cannot be overstated. But Bobby was dead, and now this. Camelot had ended.

As for *Apollo 8* on Christmas Eve—Mom's birthday—I stayed up by myself to watch the astronauts' broadcast through to the end, not long before midnight. The command module rounded the moon for the final time and, after an agonizing wait, re-established communication with Earth to announce that the engine had fired as designed, pushing them home as planned. "Houston, *Apollo 8*," said Command Pilot Jim Lovell. "Please be informed, there is a Santa Claus."

In October, however, any such thought that 1968 could be salvaged (forget end well), was an unconsidered fantasy. So I watched Smith and Carlos—on the track, on the medal stand—and breathed it all in regardless. Black was beautiful. Mysterious, scary, forbidden to a kid like me, but beautiful, too.

Home from school one afternoon and by myself, I went into the upstairs bathroom and, using my mother's eyebrow pencil, drew a goatee around my still-smooth lips and chin. I couldn't wait. This was not an unrealistic fantasy. Maybe I had the genes. Mom had been a sprinter for St. John the Evangelist Elementary back when Babe Didrikson was winning gold medals at the 1932 Los Angeles Olympics. "I loved it and I was good at it," is Mom's straightforward scouting report—at least until she collapsed on the practice field in eighth grade and, after a heart murmur diagnosis, wasn't allowed to run anymore. As for now, hadn't Norman finished second? And Larry Questad of the United States had finished sixth in that same 200 meters in the lane next to Carlos. Of course I noticed. When the Mexico flame was extinguished amid the promise of Munich and the next Quadrennial, I set out to become an African-American dash man.

I worked out four days a week, through the winter, in the mornings before school. Mondays and Fridays I took a long run, or at least what seemed like a long run then: two and a half miles up and down the Haines Acres hills. Tuesdays and Thursdays I'd run the track at York Suburban Junior High School on the edge of the Acres. Only five years old, the cinder track was already beat up and rutted, poorly maintained. It was perfect. I walked 220 yards, jogged 220, ran 220, sprinted 220, repeating it four times. I relished the 20 or 30 yards when I'd roll from one speed into the next. The churn of my legs, the thrust of my arms, the way it all grew faster and faster. I'd find my cruising speed at the new pace and lean it into the turn and down the straight until it was time to pick it up again, *go faster*. By the time I got to the 220 sprint, it was Tommie Smith, John Carlos, and me, churning our way to the victory stand. I could already envision the plaque that Springettsbury Township would erect to me here at the "Steve McKee Cinder Track."

I rarely missed an appointed day. This was my first taste of athletic success, or at least accomplishment, and I loved it. By January, I was feeling it enough to get my mouth running, too. I let it be known, not very discreetly, that I was running every morning, getting in shape, getting fast—that track season was right around the corner, and I was coming on. This popping off got me into a match race with one of the wide receivers on the football team (and hurdler on the track team). Whether he challenged me, or I him, I don't remember. By then it didn't matter.

As with all things high school, this contest came complete with its own ritual, set in stone by some unseen force. After school, we would race the length of the first-floor hallway, down and back—a good 200 yards total past all the classrooms. In our school clothes, minus the jacket, tie tucked into the shirt, cuffs of the pants rolled up once or twice. And barefoot. For verification, we would each bring witnesses.

I toed the line, my insides hollowed out by nerves. How do you run with two sockless feet in your mouth? By the end of the hallway I was a stride or two behind. We slammed into the doors of the study hall, pushed off, and headed back. I then proceeded to glide right by him, eating him up. To run on those legs just one more day! He quit at homeroom 109. I crossed the line, triumphant, at 111.

That victory got me a match race with a second football flanker, another hurdler. Same ritual, only this time down and back in the school cafeteria. I had him beat before we reached the doors. He stopped and watched, an embarrassed smile on his face, as I ran back up.

This tale now ends one of two ways. Either I tried out for the track team, went on to a state championship, a college track scholarship (at Villanova with famed coach Jumbo Elliott; it was the only place a Mid-Atlantic Catholic kid runner would choose to go), and then the Munich Olympics. Or I tried out for the team and in the early going blew everyone away, but only because I was already in shape, already running as fast as I could, and then watched as the legitimate sprinters inevitably found the higher gear that I didn't own. I reached my zenith with an early preseason win in an intrasquad 220. By the first meet of the year, against Red Lion High School, I was watching in jacket and tie, cuffs rolled down, shoes on, clothed fully in humiliation. I ran one race that season, a B-team 220, finishing second to last. I was no African-American dash man.

But that winter on the junior high track was not for naught. Not at all. I learned that I hated getting out of bed that early, but also that I could—by myself, ahead of Dad's alarm-clock cough. I discovered that when you're out there running, you own the day. I realized that I liked being in shape. That working out was just that—work—but worth it.

Also, I started seeing a dad or two from the neighborhood out there on the track, puffing around in their old Florsheims or high-top sneakers. It is generally agreed that the fitness boom in the United States officially sounded when Frank Shorter won the Munich Olympic marathon in 1972. But four years earlier, in 1968, with Dad nearly six years removed from his first attack, seeing those dads at the junior high attuned my ears to the sound of a distant rumbling.

That year Dr. Kenneth H. Cooper published *Aerobics*, a seminal tract on the benefits of exercise. I can still see the book on Mom's Early American dough-box end table in our living room. I had placed it there conspicuously in the hope that Dad would see it, read it, and get out the door himself. So yes, there was something out there warming up, stretching out, getting ready. I could feel it with every stride. Or at least I wanted to, desperately at that. I wanted Dad out there with me crunching the cinders—him and me, shoulder to shoulder. "Steve" and Steve facing up to our shared legacy while simultaneously facing it down. He had been a hunter and a fisherman all his life, but increasingly he was allowing his work to keep him from the fields and streams. I wanted him to stop smoking, eat right, quit his job. I wanted him to take charge. To get in shape, be in shape, stay in shape. He never did.

So I did it for him, and I have been doing it ever since. College basketball. Rec league hoops and volleyball. Cross-country skiing. A bicycle as primary transportation. In 1980, I returned to regular, daily running, ran a marathon, and then continued to pound out the miles until I was past forty, when the knees finally screamed in protest. I turned to a rowing machine, my 6-foot-8-inch frame well suited to the push and pull. I started lifting weights. I did nearly two years of low-impact aerobics, spent a few years ice skating, one summer swimming. I bought another bicycle. And on "off" days I walked to work at the *Wall Street Journal* in lower Manhattan, fifty minutes over the Brooklyn Bridge from our house across the East River.

Never not in shape; always the secret.

In 1990 my wife, Noreen, and I adopted a baby boy, Patrick. We were in the birthing room with his birth mother. The delivery was difficult. The ordeal left Patrick exhausted, unable even to cry for almost thirty-six hours. But when I held him in my arms for the first time and looked down at his little white stocking cap, my past, present, and future collided. Never again would I be just that sixteen-year-old kid at the junior high track trying to get his Dad in shape. I would be the father Dad never was, staying in shape for his son.

I brought all of this with me to an "executive physical" at a clinic in New Jersey on Tax Day 2005. All of it—Forjan, Dad, Patrick, the last day of my father's life, the first day of my son's. This eight hours of treadmill test, nutritional assessment, and full-body scan was not my idea. I was fifty-two years old, in shape, always had been, so what was the point? But Noreen insisted.

Once there I warmed to the task, and by the end of the day I was fairly giddy with success, ready for my Olympic gold medal, Munich 1972. Coming off the treadmill test, I was even dressed for the victory platform, in baggy sweats. I could have been running the junior high track right then. But instead I was sitting in another office with another wooden desk, now across from a cardiologist. He was affable, friendly, enthusiastic; his confidence in the technology at his disposal was unshakable. This was the second time we had talked today. Earlier, in a lengthy conversation, I had told him my story. Now he was telling me his, or at least that part about what all these various tests could reveal. He was in the business of collecting data, which could then be put to work.

Seamlessly, he turned my attention to one of the two computers on his desk. On the screen were a series of digital slides, all in shades of black and gray. Then suddenly, there it was, a blotch of white, stark in its contrast. The doctor said nothing. He didn't have to. The blockage was in about 20 percent of my left anterior descending artery. There was about the same in my right coronary artery. My risk of having a heart attack within the next twelve months: 10 percent or more, according to the data. Left untreated, the risk would only compound, making a heart attack a near certainty.

Thirty-six years melted away. Dad in the TV room, his back slammed into the couch. Coach Forjan sitting at his desk, peering at me through those horned-rim glasses. This was going to take some getting used to.

MONDAY, OCTOBER 6

Alone now. For the first time in a week—or maybe forever—Mom and Kathy and I were by ourselves. No sitting with Nana in the parlor of her house on Rodney Avenue, sunk deep into the scrunchy mohair cushions of an ancient maroon sofa, barely able to see over its lace-doily arms. No living room full of relatives at Aunt Evie's house in Hamburg, New York, south of Buffalo. No house full of friends in York, people coming and going with food and drink or bringing my green herringbone suit back from the cleaners so it would be ready for the viewing. No one just hanging around from the "York Crowd," Mom and Dad's close circle, everyone in it transferred to York from someplace else over the past fifteen years or so, only by accident winding up in East York and St. Joseph Church.

No, we were alone now. Over the weekend we had returned Dad to Buffalo, and earlier this morning we had returned to York. The house seemed bigger. Or our family seemed smaller. Something. Nothing needed to be done, no arrangements made. It was over. Now what?

"Oh, my God, I can't believe he saved this," Mom said. She had emptied Dad's personal effects from a York Hospital envelope onto the dining room table. I don't remember all the contents, but here is an excellent guess. A half-used roll of Tums. Dad loved his Tums. He believed in Tums. Calcium carbonate cured all ills, except maybe denial. The week before his first heart attack, in 1963, complaining of pain in his chest—indigestion, it had to be—he had turned to his Tums and a nap until the crisis had passed. The very day of his attack the next week, he counted on his Tums to see him through—until they couldn't.

There were also probably a couple of salt pills on the table. Dad loved his salt pills, too; always a handful with a gulp of water before heading out to mow the lawn. His wedding ring would have spun onto the tablecloth. It was a nondescript, thin platinum band, with the date—November 8, 1947—etched inside if not still readable. An inexpensive watch, his ten-year award from Cole Steel Equipment Company; a set of car keys inside a folded brown-leather case; a worn rosary. Probably about 81 cents in loose change, a Zippo lighter for sure, and (unless he'd put them on the end table next to the sofa in the TV room Tuesday night) the omnipresent pack of cigarettes.

There was also his wallet, a beat-up old brown. It was a particular bit of its contents that had brought forth Mom's I-can't-believe-it. I was sitting across from her at the table. It was one of her prize possessions, this table, an Early American replica antique of soft dark pine. It nicked and bruised easily, and Kathy and I had learned to tread carefully around it. Once, after doing something wrong that I have now forgotten, I had to write out my punishment multiple times on a piece of paper.

Mom must not have been around because I sat at this table with paper and pen, etching "I shall not . . . I shall not . . . I shall not . . ." into the wood, where it remained for years until Mom finally had the table refinished.

Mom carefully unfolded a worn and yellowed piece of writing paper. Even from across the table I could recognize her handwriting on it. "It's a letter I wrote to your father when he was in the South Pacific during the war."

Mom said she couldn't believe it, but she probably did. Dad was a packrat of the first order. *Don't throw it out!* If it was old, save it. Once, he returned from a day's fishing with the game pocket zippered onto the back of his jacket stuffed not with trout but with a giant stack of order forms, dated to the 1940s, from some now-forgotten company. Where he'd found them, I don't know; how they had survived, who knows. But he couldn't have been happier had he come home with the Big One. He kept those order forms in the garage for years.

Mom read the letter to herself. Dad had joined the Army Air Corps in January 1943 and wasn't mustered out and back in Buffalo until January 1946. By then Mom was in Germany with the War Department, a secretary at the Nuremberg War Crimes Trial for another four months. I watched as she tried to hold herself together. She couldn't. Her hands started to shake, her lips to tremble, and then she burst into tears, a violent wail, her emotions overflowing beyond her for the first time all week.

When you're a kid, the story of how your parents created the union that eventually created you seems a necessary part of the natural order, fated, as etched in stone as the Ten Commandments. Even when you learn it isn't, when you discover its utter capriciousness, you don't believe it. You can't.

Mom and Dad met in the summer of 1938, out at Sunset Bay, a tiny triangle of a lakeshore spot in Chautauqua County, framed by Lake Erie, some railroad tracks, and Cattaraugus Creek. The beach is said to be the best on the U.S. side of the lake. With Dad from East Buffalo and Mom from South, there seems no way that their lives would have intersected up in the city. They met, officially, at a place on Iola Drive called Town Hall, the cottage Dad shared with his East Buffalo buddies, named in honor of the popular Fred Allen radio show, "Town Hall Tonight." If there was magic in the moment, it was Dad who recognized it. Growing up, Kathy and I never heard about Dad's having other girlfriends. Because for Dad, from the beginning, Mom was the one and only. "He was never obvious about it," Aunt Alice says. "But I think he just made up his mind: this is it."

Dad spent his high school years and a first year of preparation at the Minor Seminary of the Buffalo Roman Catholic Diocese. His class graduation picture shows Dad in the back row, in dark suit with boutonniere, his hair uncharacteristically askew. He graduated in 1936 and then left in 1937 after the college prep year, when he was required to make a longer-term commitment. Turning his back on the priesthood broke Nana's heart in that old-fashioned, irreparable, Irish Catholic way. And then Dad met Mom. He was nineteen; she, seventeen.

As for Mom and that Town Hall fortuity, she remembers nothing of it, even as she allows how destined it all seems now.

She shrugs her shoulders: they met. She was with her girl-friends; he was with his guys.

Mom and Dad had "their" song—"I'll Never Smile Again" by the Tommy Dorsey Band, sung by a Frank Sinatra whose most prominent feature was still his Adam's apple. When Dad took me and Kathy and Mom out to dinner on special occasions, it was my job to excuse myself discreetly (I thought) to ask the organist or piano player if he knew the song. Back at the table I'd sit with barely contained anticipation, keyed to the tune, watching Mom for that glistening look of recognition that never failed to materialize. "I'll Never Smile Again." Today when I hear it—rarely, making it all the more out-of-nowhere—the song is an arrow right through me, carrying me back to a 1938, a Lake Erie, a *that moment* of my imagination. Except the song wasn't written until 1939, by the Canadian-American songwriter Ruth Lowe of Toronto (across Lake Ontario from Buffalo, at least) and the Dorsey-Sinatra Victor recording wasn't a big hit until the summer of 1940—a good two years past that Sunset Bay, Town Hall night.

Kathy and I always knew that for Mom there had been other beaux. More than a few, in fact. Dad hadn't been the only guy Mom had written to during the war. And it's not that she talked about any of them very much. She didn't. We just knew. (This was not the least bit upsetting to us; indeed, just the opposite. Through it all, despite it all, Dad had won out, creating our destiny.) One was the son of a judge, one of thirteen kids. "We were pretty serious," Mom says. "At least I thought I was. Or, I thought we were. I know *he* was."

But far and away the most famous of Mom's formers in the McKee household was a man with a long, three-part German name, twenty-two letters long if I am spelling it correctly. He was the man Mom likely was dating when she and Dad met. They may have been engaged. Mom rarely mentioned him, though when she did it was with obvious remembered affection. We never learned why it didn't work out (what could she tell us?); in fact we learned very little about him. It was Kathy and I who kept him alive. We delighted in saying his name, a real mouthful. We'd trip all over it, laughing. Then Kathy would say to me, "You would have been Hansel!" And I'd answer back, "You would have been Gretel!" And we'd laugh some more.

He is, Mom believes, still alive. It would be most ungentlemanly of me to include his name here. In 1991, after the funeral of Leo Callaghan, the husband of Aunt Marg, Mom's oldest sister, we repaired to Stan's, Uncle Leo's Friday-night fish-fry Buffalo-Polish taproom of choice. Mom called me aside and said, "I'd like you to meet someone." She then turned to the man next to her. This, Mom said, is . . . *the man with the three-part German name*. He was a card-playing pal of Uncle Leo's. For the first time ever, there was nothing hilariously infectious about his moniker. There he was, right in front of me. Not terribly tall. Fastidiously dressed. Natty blue blazer. Bow-tied. Clipped gray mustache. A certain formal bearing. So completely, utterly, totally . . . not Dad. I understood immediately that Mom was introducing me to more than just a former beau. I was shaking hands with a piece of her life that I could never really know. Even more, I was meeting a life that for her had never happened—and if it had, it would have meant no life for me.

But Mom and Dad had happened, and because they had I was here now, sitting across the dining room table as Mom wept for the life that she and Dad had made. She may have written to other men during the war, but she was crying for only one of them now. She was forty-eight years old, married for less than twenty-two years. To me, in that moment those numbers seemed immutable and forever, so implacably timeless I probably gave them no thought at all. Mom and Dad, they just always were. Now this stuns me. All of it taken by a heart attack.

The outburst at the dining room table over the letter forgotten by Mom but remembered by Dad caught me completely unawares, utterly defenseless. And so it began, and for the rest of my life: when my mother cries, I cry too.

I cannot possibly overplay the significance of this next sentence. Without Mom, I would not have survived that first year after Dad died. It is impossible for me to imagine how I could have, in a scenario that isn't dominated by her. It is an emotion that remained for me right beneath the skin, for years and years difficult to talk about, even think about. That I finally got over it I credit, of all people, a seven-year-old Patrick McKee.

In February 1998, Mom, then seventy-seven, faced triple-bypass surgery with possible valve replacement. (As with women and coronary artery disease, Mom's had arrived pretty much on schedule.) I took Patrick with me to York beforehand for a weekend, to lend some support but mainly to tell her, finally, the one thing, the only thing, that had to be said. I put off telling her as long as I could, of course. Then, with the weekend dwindling and opportunity passing, I ensconced Patrick in front of the TV upstairs, cranked the volume, closed the door, and went down to the kitchen. Now or maybe never.

After a long windup I finally released. I didn't need to tell her I loved her, though I told her so. I needed to tell her how grateful I was that she had been so tough, so unbelievably tough, in those first few months, the first year, the rest of my life, after Dad died. That's what I needed to tell her, what she needed to hear, just in case. How she had refused to break, refused even to bend. Day after day she kept it going, kept it together. Had she not, I would have been lost, and I sometimes think forever. The words, twenty-nine years in the coming, hacked from me now in breath-choking gags, my arms splayed out in front of me on the kitchen table for balance, my fists clenched.

Then the phone rang.

This is the Springettsbury Township Police. The same department that in 1969 had radioed for an ambulance to Stanford Drive. *Can you confirm a nine-one-one call made from this number?* The question came so completely from nowhere, penetrated so deeply into a space where it didn't belong, that I had no idea what to say except the obvious: "Nine-one-one?" Then suddenly Patrick materialized from around the corner at the end of the hall. He stood there almost paralyzed, curly blond hair framing the fearful look on his face. Two plus two quickly became four. He had heard me—up the stairs and over the TV—gotten scared and called the cops, likely hanging up as soon as he heard someone talk-ing. "It's okay, officer, no problem here," I said. And there wasn't, not anymore. I can tell Mom anything now; she's nearly eighty-seven, no time for important thoughts to be left unsaid. "Nine-one-one, Mom," is all I have to say. Tension breaks before it is built, and off I go.

One story of Mom from those early months. The Christmas vacation had started, and I was off from York Catholic. On her way to work she corralled me in the foyer. "We are going to celebrate Christmas this year," she said. "And we are going to enjoy it." There was more. "By the time I get home tonight, you will have put up the Christmas tree and you will have dec-orated it." So very Mom, employing the precise verb tense. This was the last thing I wanted to be doing that day, any day. But I went through the familiar motions, bringing up the bar-rel with the Christmas stuff, its dusty, evocative smell casting none of its usual spell, then the stand and the lights. I dragged in the tree from out back. Mr. Schmitt and Mr. Leahy, two York Crowd regulars, had taken me out the weekend before to pick it out.

I got the tree up, into the stand, lights on, and moved it into the traditional corner. But when I backed up for a look, the tree was listing awkwardly. I crawled underneath on my belly to tighten and loosen screws. That's when the tree fell over, right on top of me. I had just enough time to tuck myself into a fetal position, and that's where I stayed, buried in Douglas fir (we always got a Douglas fir), bawling my eyes out for a few minutes until I could stand the heat of the lights no longer. But when Mom got home from work, the Christmas tree was up, perpendicular to the floor, and decorated. The McKees celebrated Christmas in 1969, and we enjoyed it. Mom had said so.

She came by her toughness, that independence, honestly. In May 1933, Mom's mother, Agnes, died mysteriously, or at least puzzlingly, at Mercy Hospital in Buffalo. Mystery and puzzlement because even though her death certificate fairly clearly lays out events, Mom has always felt that there was more to the story than what the family had been told. Agnes had entered the hospital on May 8 for a hysterectomy. She died eight days later, cause of death "peritonitis, postoperative" of six days' duration. But Mom remembers that her mother went into the hospital for the operation, came home, and then went back in. She says that a few years later she and her older sister, Evelyn, attempted to piece together what happened. A plausible if unknowable scenario is that Agnes went in for an exploratory procedure, but once she was on the operating table doctors discovered a cancer of some sort. They had sent her home, telling her little and the family less, knowing that she had only weeks. When she returned and they operated, she died on the table. That's all they were told. Mom believes that her mother may have bled to death during the operation. Agnes Marie Bunce O'Neil was forty-four years old.

Agnes's husband, my grandfather, was Andrew O'Neil, forty-five years old in 1933. They had married on June 27, 1910. Agnes, a telephone operator before she wed, was active in the politics of the Old First Ward, a regular at the polls on Election Day. Agnes and Andy together enjoyed "an active so-

cial life," Mom recalls, regularly entertaining friends or going
to friends' homes. They also enjoyed the picture shows at the
Maxine Theater at the end of Seneca Parkside, where it runs
into Seneca Street. They had four children: Margaret (who
turned twenty-two the May that Agnes died), Evelyn (seventeen), Andrew (fifteen), and Helen (twelve). For years when
his kids were little, Andy worked as a conductor for the New
York Central or Nickel Plate railroads. He apparently made
good money, when there was money to be made. A switch-
man's strike in 1920 proved especially bountiful. When Helen
Teresa O'Neil was born at St. Mary's Maternity Hospital on
Christmas Eve that year, Andy came back to Seneca Parkside
through a sixteen-degree night and hastily put up the Christmas tree for the three other kids, festooning it with the most
readily available decoration—a blizzard of dollar bills he tied
to the branches.

Mom traipsed Kathy and me up to Buffalo from York every
summer when we were kids. I say "traipsed," but I loved it.
The crowded weeklong itinerary always included some sequence of Dad's side at Rodney Avenue, where Nana lived on
the first floor and Aunt Mary Jane and Uncle Chuck Gampp
lived with their six kids on the second. I got to sleep in the attic, Dad's old bedroom, staring up at the peeling cowboy-and-
Indian wallpaper. The seven Clarence Center cousins (the kids
of Aunt Alice and Uncle Bob Murphy, east of Buffalo) would
always come to visit if we didn't go out there. And then we'd
be off to Mom's two sisters—Marg in Lakeview and Ev in
Hamburg. There were also usually visits with Mom's two favored cousins, George Engler and Jack Reedy—brothers who

were raised as cousins, their once-lost, then-found story a defining family drama. There were tears every year when we got into the car for the drive back to York.

Where we didn't go was to Andy O'Neil's house. It was never on the regular tour. Surely that's why it is Dad's Rodney Avenue, and not Mom's Seneca Parkside, that still resonates for me. I remember being at Andy's house once in all of our Buffalo summers. He lived with a couple of old ladies, though I never knew exactly who they were. Thinking about it now, there must have been Buffalo visits when Mom didn't go see him at all. I have only one strong memory of him—we grandkids, Peter and Denny Callaghan and I, surrounding him in a chair—though it is likely that I remember it at all because we have a snapshot.

Even as a kid I understood there was something wrong with this picture. That there was something between Mom and her father; something between all three O'Neil sisters and Andy O'Neil. Years later, in 1976 at a family wedding, Peter Callaghan, then a Franciscan priest who had performed the ceremony, started asking questions of all three sisters. *What was the deal with Andy after your mother died?* The reception was over and we had continued the festivities at the hotel. The Montreal Summer Olympics were on TV, and I was listening to an interview with Frank Shorter explaining his silver-medal finish behind East Germany's Waldemar Cierpinski in the marathon when Peter started in. *There was something. All us kids could tell.* Peter knew, too? Silently I egged him on, even as his questions clearly backed all three sisters uncomfortably against a wall, none of them wanting to answer.

And then all of a sudden Mom, the baby of the family, in no uncertain words declared the subject off limits. Period. Her unvarnished truth, filled with unresolved pain, left me slacked-jawed. Many years later I asked Mom if she remembered this. She said she didn't. But neither did she deny that it could have happened.

Andy O'Neil—an affable, lovable Irishman, to hear tell—came apart after Agnes died. That appears to be the gist of it. She had been holding him together, holding the family together, most likely, and after she passed the girls were on their own. He was there but he wasn't there. He'd play bingo after work, then come home and eat peanut butter crackers and drink beer at the kitchen table. He died in 1961. Mom was at his bedside; the three sisters had been taking turns keeping vigil. Mom says that by the end the rough edges had been smoothed, reconciliations made, by all of them. "Looking back, I realize my father wasn't all that bad," Mom says. She searched for a pleasant remembrance. Turns out he was a regular at Buffalo's boxing matches—as often as not with a very young Mom in tow. (Agnes would not have approved!) He took her to baseball games, too: the Buffalo Bisons finished first in the International League in 1936 before losing the Little World Series to the Milwaukee Brewers. She loved both, if only because they provided her time with her father. And Mom says, "He held a job"—no small consideration, given the times. "He just couldn't cope."

In any event, only with Agnes gone could the great family legend of the Famous O'Neil Sisters commence. (That's what Kathy and I called Marg, Ev, and Helen, with both genuine affection and next-generation sarcasm.) Franklin Delano Roosevelt had been sworn in as president only two months before. Fear itself lurked, despite the new president's implorings. In 1933, Buffalo marked its centennial. The city owed its existence to the Erie Canal, but that had opened in 1825 and its time had long passed.

Aunts Nell, Rose, and Margaret, Andy's three maiden sisters (the semimysterious old ladies of my summer visit) moved in with them. Mom's sister Marg worked at Abbott Lumber and brought money home. Ev was a student at State Teachers. Mom was in sixth grade, wanting nothing more than to attend Mount Mercy Academy on Red Jacket Parkway on the other side of Cazenovia Park and then go off to college herself. (She reached Mount Mercy, but much to a long regret, not beyond it. Ev worked the soda counter at Parsons & Judd Drugstore to get Mom through the secretarial course at Hurst's Private School.) Mom's assignment in the meantime was to come home from school and make dinner. Andy would give her a dollar to buy groceries. When she needed instructions she would yell through the kitchen window to "Aunt Josie" next door, across a narrow driveway. If Mom needed an ingredient or two, Aunt Josie could pass it to her through the windows on the flat end of a broom. This was no small stretch: the houses on Seneca Parkside, a one-block-long street ending at the park, are separated by a good nine feet of driveway.

This was their life—more or less, or at least in the telling—until 1940, when Aunt Marg married Leo Callaghan, a twenty-five-year-old policeman. Eight years for Mom to do all her growing up, from twelve to twenty. Eight years for the Famous

O'Neil Sisters to grow intensely close and remain so forever, through all the joy and sadness and inevitable sorority aggravations of the rest of their lives. They practiced the forgotten art of letter writing—for years and years, one or two a week passed from each to the other—and what I wouldn't give for them to have saved every one, our family history recounted in everyday detail.

Surprisingly, or perhaps not, what happened to Mom—the early death of a parent; the surviving spouse irreversibly jolted by it—had happened to Andy. His mother had died in 1891, when he was seven years old. Margaret Brady was born in Drumcho, County Cavan, Ireland, in 1845, the second oldest of at least ten children. The story is that when she was about twenty she came to America on the *Great Eastern*, the ship that put down the first successful transatlantic telegraph cable. She settled in New York City, but while watching a parade up in Albany she had recognized James O'Neil, from Drumcho. They married and eventually moved to Buffalo, where James drove a truck for Brady Brothers Lumber, owned by a couple of Margaret's brothers. She died after contracting pneumonia while attending a family funeral in a rainstorm. James, in his early fifties by then, chose not to recover. Andy was the youngest of the six surviving children. In his turn, he would have twenty years to observe his father's grief before James died. Back from his day at the lumber company, James would send one of his kids to the pub across the street to have his lunch pail filled with beer. It is said he was given to singing the popular song "When You and I Were Young, Maggie."

So now it was Mom's turn. Agnes hadn't died so a twelve-year-old Mom would know how to perform—or how not to—when in 1969 she would become a forty-eight-year-old widow herself. Yet in the uncanny way that family generations spill one onto the next, revisiting, reinventing, repeating themselves, that's what happened. Sitting there at the dining room table, reading a wartime letter she'd forgotten she wrote to a sentimental packrat in the South Pacific who always remembered, I believe Mom understood that her moment had arrived. She could choose now to recover, or not. Kathy and I kid about how for us the international indicator that Mom has determined her course of action (and we should just surrender to it) is a thinning of her lips and a squaring of her jaw. I can't say I saw Mom do that on that Monday morning. But as sure as I am that Dad died with 81 cents in his pocket, I know that's how Mom looked at me across the table, in a house much bigger than it used to feel. The outcome was never in doubt.

SATURDAY, OCTOBER 4

THE SERVICE BY THE GRAVESIDE WAS OVER. MUCH OF THE BUF-
falo weekend was over. My first airplane ride yesterday. The
viewing last night, where I met Dad's friends from the old
days, the ones he had always talked so much about, telling me
the stories of when he was a kid growing up. Jack Nussbaum in
particular, Dad's loyalest boyhood buddy. Best man at his wedding. During the war they had even been stationed not far
from each other in the South Pacific, Dad, with the 1062nd
Quartermaster Corps, Jack, with a B-25 group. Two boys from
Buffalo in the middle of all that. Jack Nussbaum had always
loomed large in Dad's recountings. Now here he was, looming
large right in front of me—big, powerful, a broad nose, a full
head of wavy hair, still blond.

The Requiem Mass was at Blessed Trinity, Dad's boyhood
church, a stunning homage to the architecture of the Lom-
bardy region of northern Italy in the twelfth century. In the
1970s it would be nominated to the National Register of His-
toric Places. I researched that, but Dad had even told stories

of this. Its groundbreaking had been in 1923, the dedication in 1928. From his desk in the parish's elementary school, Dad, grade by grade, had watched the church go up, brick by brick. And at Blessed Trinity Roman Catholic Church on Leroy Avenue in Buffalo, New York, it is about the bricks—misshapened, unmolded chunks in mismatched shades of red and black arranged in fabulous patterns on walls two feet thick. Workmen crawling everywhere with mortar and wheelbarrows. With a view to all that, Dad would ask me, how was an eight-year-old supposed to pay attention in school? Indeed, his Blessed Trinity stories usually came at the end of a lecture on how I needed to pay attention in school, as if to let me know he understood he was asking the impossible.

But that was over now, the Mass and the shrieking of the woman singing in the balcony, her voice fingernails across a blackboard. We talk about her to this day. We thank her, really, for the moment when Kathy and I glanced at each other and Mom bent close, stifling a laugh and whispering out loud what we were thinking: "Thank God your father's dead, because he'd go up in the balcony and strangle her." It shattered the tension, if only for an instant, as surely as a lumpy brick through a stained-glass window.

I turned from the grave and walked, not even sure I was walking the right way. I had to walk. A light touch on my right elbow turned me a bit, but I didn't break stride. It was Mr. Masterson, another of my parents' friends—Dad had taught him to fly-fish—who had moved to York from someplace else, joined St. Joseph Church, and put down roots. The shared story, the common bond, it had now brought the Baulers,

Flicks, Mastersons, McEntees, Philbins, and Schmitts up from York to bury Dad in Buffalo.

Mr. and Mrs. Masterson were late arrivals to York, coming from Chicago with five kids when I was in sixth grade. Two more would be born in York. He has the kind of sense of humor where in a crowd you need to stick close by or you'll miss out. Dad thoroughly enjoyed his company. So did I. He was one of the dads from the neighborhood whom I had started to see down at the junior high track in the mornings my junior year, making those first tentative stabs at getting in shape, reclaiming themselves. As with a couple of the York dads, he had been out of town on Tuesday, on business, their absence adding more uncertainty to the night. In fact, he had just now arrived, barely making the cemetery. I wanted to turn and fall into his arms and cry on his shoulder. I should have. But I didn't. I couldn't. I had to keep walking.

I have been to my father's Buffalo gravesite exactly once, the day I walked away. For years I didn't even know the name of the cemetery. I discovered it almost by mistake when paging through the registry book of Dad's two-night wake. A total of 418 people came to the viewings, one in York on Thursday, the other in Buffalo on Friday. There is a running tally in parentheses on some of the pages, in what I'd wager is my sixteen-year-old handwriting. The Buffalo wake was bolstered by a full contingent of sisters from St. Francis Hospital, where Nana worked as a switchboard operator. Numbers like this mattered to me in that moment. I remember turning around in the limousine on the way to the cemetery to count the following cars.

Dad's boyhood house at 231 Rodney Avenue no longer exists. Nana died in 1978, and Aunt Mary Jane, who had lived there all her life, sold the place in 1980. There was a fire at some point, and the owners in 1994 filed a permit to "demolish to grade a 2 story frame 1 family dwling." The narrow lot, the only open space on the block, is just weeds. The clapboard houses on Dad's side of the street are a bit worn, but most of the ones across the street are painted and well kept. Until a recent visit, the last time I had been there was the summer of 1978, after I got married in York and my wife, Noreen, and I stopped in Buffalo to see Nana on our way back to Alaska, where we lived from 1975 to 1982.

I parked the car this time and walked the block, the emptiness at 231 tugging at me. When Mom had brought Kathy and me up here every summer, she turned the car left from Hill Street onto Rodney, and we'd strain to find Nana's place, down on the left. Mom pulled the car into the narrow driveway between the houses. "This driveway gets skinnier every year!" Mom would exclaim, the official beginning of our Buffalo stay. This time, a shout from a neighboring porch wanted to know if I was "with the city." Another asked if I was a "real-estate man." *No, my dad used to live here . . . hadn't been back . . . just wanted to see.* This wasn't Dad's neighborhood anymore, nor mine from those boyhood visits. It belonged to other people now, people with the experience to wonder why some white guy was walking their block, poking around.

My point here is that when up in Buffalo, I go back to Rodney Avenue. Where I don't go is Dad's grave. And while that is not on purpose, it is no accident, either.

After Andy O'Neil died, and well before Dad's fatal heart attack in 1969, I once asked Mom if she planned to visit her Dad's grave when we were next up in Buffalo. "No!" she said, her answer tackling my question. Then she told me this story. After her mother died, her father regularly dragged the family to the cemetery, where he would sit by the grave and weep, wrecking another potentially pleasant Sunday afternoon for his youngest daughter. "I promised myself right then," Mom said, "that when I was old enough to decide for myself, I would never, ever visit a cemetery again." Her vow made sense to me, even then.

We took Dad back to Buffalo to bury him because . . . well, because why? Dad had fled Buffalo as soon as he could after World War II, and he never looked back at the "Queen City of the Lakes." Even as a kid I understood there was meaning in that.

He was born on January 21, 1919, at Buffalo Women's Hospital on Georgia Street, into a Buffalo with its best days likely behind it. In 1901, President William McKinley had been assassinated at the Pan American Exposition bordering Buffalo's Delaware Park, the grand Frederick Law Olmsted landscape about eight blocks west of Rodney Avenue. The exposition, called Rainbow City because its buildings were festooned in shades of red, blue, green, and gold, had opened that spring in the optimistic glow of hundreds of thousands of electric light bulbs powered by the generators at Niagara Falls. The centerpiece was the 375-foot Electric Tower, a deep green trimmed in cream, white, blue, and gold. With its 40,000-plus light bulbs, it was declared that the tower could be seen from downtown! Here was the future, switched on, and its home address was Buffalo, New York, USA, *the World*. Then in September two gunshots from the anarchist (and quite possibly mentally ill) Leon Czolgosz killed both the president and the promise. The exposition limped to a close, the assassin executed—by electric power.

Dad's boyhood seems to have been almost idyllic, at least in the telling he gave it. The house at 231, on the East Side, was about ten years old when the McKees bought it in 1922. Dad was three years old. Prior to that they had been renting on the Lower West Side, closer to the water and downtown, a few blocks from the half-finished Immaculate Conception Church where Dad had been baptized. In truth, that house has more to recommend it than does the nondescript Rodney. A sprawling, turreted three-story, it boasts charm and character, tucked well off the street. The lot next door is empty now, but were there buildings, the front door would be reachable only by a long, private walkway. Perhaps that's why there is rumor of the place having once been a brothel. Leaving that neighborhood, where Nana had grown up and Jack had taken a room at a boardinghouse, surely had to have been a major move. But at 231, the McKees *owned*. Jack, thirty-three, and the former Anna Carey, twenty-seven, brought three children with them—Thomas Francis (four), John Joseph, Jr., and Edward (twenty-two months). Mary Jane and Alice Elizabeth, originally Helen Kathryn but changed at the insistence of Nana's mother, came home to Rodney in the Novembers of 1922 and 1923, respectively.

There would be one great sadness. Edward died on September 14, 1927, at age seven. The death certificate states "ruptured appendix" as the cause. Today penicillin would most surely have cured this. The certificate records an operation two days before, and there remains in the family a whisper that the real cause of death was botched anesthesia. There can be no way to know, of course, and no one was talking about it then. But coupled with Mom's still wondering if perhaps her mother, Agnes, might have bled to death during *her* operation, it seems, if nothing else, that there are lessons to be gleaned from the perils of a less forthcoming age.

Item 14 on Edward's death certificate reads: THE ABOVE IS TRUE TO THE BEST OF MY KNOWLEDGE. Beneath is the signature *John J. McKee.* I look at the penmanship and I see my grandfather, pen in hand, and in this moment he comes fully alive to me. His dark wavy hair. The kindly face I have seen in the few photographs. He is no longer the impersonal "Jack McKee" or "my grandfather" or "Dad's dad." He is what we grandkids never got to call him: "Grand Pop" or "Pop-Pop" or "Nono" or who knows what. Standing there inconsolable, he was probably in shirt and tie. Aunt Alice says he was always in shirt and tie, even at work beneath the overalls, even at home when washing the car. And surely he was when they dressed Edward in his white First Communion suit, waked him from 231, and then took him to Blessed Trinity for the Requiem Mass.

Immediately to the west and north of Rodney Avenue are the neighborhoods of Parkside and Central Park. Parkside is home to a Frank Lloyd Wright complex, in the architect's Prairie Style. Central Park was developed by Lewis J. Bennett of the Bennett Cement Company, who, it is said, had walked the streets himself telling a blaster where to dynamite holes to plant the elm trees that would grace the area for decades. He built the foundations for his homes using black-flecked Onondaga limestone that he mined from the Bennett Quarry—across a wide and dividing Main Street in Dad's Fillmore-Leroy neighborhood just north of the three-block Rodney. I have found a single instance of this area being called the "Valley of the Tears." That is telling, perhaps. As anecdotally explained to me, it could be a German reference to the late Teens and early 1920s, when the Irish started moving in, pushing out the longtime Teutons. Those Irish, of course, would have included the McKees, whose Lower West Side was becoming more Italian. Whatever the truth, Rodney wasn't part of Parkside, nor of Central Park. But Rodney did have the quarry.

The quarry! If I seem obsessed with it, it's because I am, because Dad was. Like 231 Rodney, the quarry is gone now. Urban development filled in the area's distinguishing landmark in the early 1950s, replacing it with the Central Park Plaza, a parking lot currently bordered by a boarded-up strip mall. But the Bennett Quarry lived in Dad's remembering and lives now in my imagining. He loved to talk about being a kid, with best buddies Jack Nausbaum and Joe Folkman, heading straight to the pit after school, or lollygagging there all day long in the summer. He could tell a great story, Dad could, and he made it all sound like great adventure. They spent all their free time there, climbing the rocks, catching rabbits in homemade snares, swimming in the summer, ice skating in the winter. There were fossils to be found there, too. When they got hungry they foraged for tubers, built a fire, and cooked them up, using the flames to dry out their clothes before going home for dinner, stinking of smoke and boyhood.

That your parent had once been a kid, that's beyond the ken. Dad used to talk about how he never owned a store-bought bicycle. He and his buddies built them from found objects in the neighborhood, the quarry being the local dumping ground as well. This I could never believe. He built bicycles from scrap? And then he *rode* them? Dad on a bike, I couldn't see it. Then one Christmas, Kathy and I both got bikes (mine black and silver, heavy with fenders and fuselage, an early-1960s beauty; Kathy's the girl's model in royal blue and white). Dad put them together himself the night before, of course, and then in the morning, before he let us take them out, he hopped aboard and tested them down Wilshire Drive, where we lived in way-out East York till I was in the sixth grade and we moved closer in to Haines Acres. Dad on a bike! It couldn't have been more of a shock had he been riding a stagecoach down the street.

Dad could fix anything. Or at least he thought he could. Or at least he would try to. Some of that he likely got from his dad. As a plasterer, Jack probably had his hands in some of Buffalo's biggest construction projects in the 1920s and 1930s. Buffalo's City Hall, a spectacular thirty-two-story Art Deco edifice overlooking Lake Erie, was dedicated in 1932. And we do know he worked on the Hotel Statler, the grand palace on Niagara Square downtown; it opened in 1923. Perhaps he also worked the interior of Blessed Trinity, though I think Dad would have told me that. And on Rodney Avenue he took out the inside entrance door, along with an entire wall, and replaced it with an archway of his own design.

Jack had three brothers and four sisters. The brothers—William, Frank, and Edward—also worked the trades. Growing up in northeast Pennsylvania, it was go into a trade or go into the mines, and their mother insisted they not go into the mines. Her father had. Frank and Edward often bunked at Rodney Avenue, sometimes for extended periods, when there was work to be found in western New York. Aunt Alice says that the McKee kids always knew when to expect a visit: in the days before, Jack McKee took to singing "She'll Be Coming 'Round the Mountain." Dad was quite close to Uncle Ed, and Uncle Frank shows up on the 1930 census as both plumber and Rodney resident. What Jack didn't teach Dad, these uncles likely did. Including, unavoidably, death by heart attack. The dozen years beginning with Jack McKee's probable coronary occlusion on July 6, 1941, were not kind to the sons of Frank and Mary Ann McKee of Oak Street in North Scranton, the old Providence area. Edward died of a coronary thrombosis in 1945 at age forty-three; Frank of an acute coronary in 1948 at fifty; William of an acute coronary thrombosis in 1953, at least at sixty-three the longest-lived brother.

Getting his hands dirty made Dad happy—under the hood, down in the basement, beneath the sink—followed by a good hard washing with a bar of Lava soap. In 1957, Dad and Mom bought a three-and-a-half-acre farm farther out in East York for $8,000, one of the parcels of land owned by the Witmer family, a longtime York County clan. Ramshackle house, huge barn, a few outbuildings, everything was in constant need of repair, both major and minor. Dad loved his time at the farm—fixing, cleaning; cleaning, fixing. He laid new tile, put in new electrical. He brought the bathroom into the house; when they bought the place there was a plumbed toilet out in the chicken coop. Dad was no craftsman, but he got it done. He also enjoyed getting himself out past where he knew what he was doing. There was challenge in that, and if it meant another trip to the hardware store, what was so bad about that? Sometimes we'd make two, three trips on a Saturday.

I loved going with him to the farm, spending the time with him, keeping a wrench on the nut while he tightened the bolt, that sort of thing. It was me who figured out how to cut the new plastic shower wall around the bathroom fixtures. Though it's the fuss Dad made over it that night at dinner that I remember. But the fact is I never got it, I never understood the appeal. There was always something—leaky faucet, balky furnace, sagging floorboard—that inevitably brought forth from Dad a blue-streaked oath. He could swear with the best of them (though I didn't first hear the F-word from him), and he was at his most creative out there at the farm.

Once I called him on it. I asked him why. Why did he bother with the farm, why did he and Mom own it, put themselves through this? It all seemed like such a burden, a waste of time. He looked at me like I had a screw loose, only this one he couldn't make tight. The realization pained him. The disconnect between us was large. He pulled out the stock, completely true reply: the farm was our college education. What he didn't tell me—if I was asking the question I wouldn't understand the answer—was that he loved everything about it, trying to keep it going until such time as he and Mom needed it. Everything, up to and including when the wrench slipped, his knuckles got scraped, and the swearing began.

I still believe his penchant to fix-it-myself helped him along to his first heart attack. In the autumn of 1962, Dad declared it was time to finish our cinder-block basement on Wilshire Drive, turn it into the classic 1950s-style rec room with cork-tile floor, knotty-pine paneling, and tile ceiling. The room proved too damp for paneling (and the paneling probably too expensive), but the rest Dad set about installing. He started by renting a belt sander to remove the green paint from the cement floor. He spent a Saturday enveloped in a Dust Bowl cloud, then came up for dinner. "Let's see how I'm doing," he declared enthusiastically, standing in the kitchen layered in dirt. He pulled out a handkerchief and blew his nose, then triumphantly showed us a great green gob that used to be the basement floor. Dad's next project had begun.

Laying the cork tile proved straightforward. The tongue-and-groove ceiling was another matter. It was no easy-install drop canopy. First Dad had to level the beams that lined the open ceiling with shims and slats, then create a lattice work at right angles to the beams, leveling them as he went. Only then could he start tacking up the foot-square beige tiles one by one. For months he spent an hour or two in the evening after work tap-tap-tapping away, arms above his shoulders, head back, neck straining. He was in the basement when it happened. He decided to take a break, chew a few Tums, lie down for a while.

————

When Dad was born in 1919, Jack and Anna McKee could reasonably have expected their second baby boy to live until he was about fifty-six years old. Cause of death, using the statistics of the day, pneumonia or influenza. Those were no idle threat. Buffalo's population had grown nearly 20 percent between 1910 and 1920, to more than half a million people, but the great influenza of 1918 had hit the city hard. Buffalo was a significant inland port of entry, and through it poured the so-called Spanish flu. For a time, the city itself was in the coffin-making business because private contractors couldn't meet demand. Worldwide, the death toll was staggering, surely beyond Jack's and Anna's comprehension. Even today there is no final count: fifty million people isn't conservative. Weld any such number to the killing machine that was World War I, ended barely two months when Dad was born, and it's safe to assume that for Mr. and Mrs. John McKee, "atherosclerosis" was not on their worry list.

Perhaps it should have been. "Diseases of the heart" had occupied the top spot as the leading cause of death in the United States since at least 1910, save for the three influenza years of 1918, 1919, and 1920. Ironically, part of what was happening here was that people were finally living long enough for heart disease to manifest its deadly characteristic.

That same year of 1919, Dr. James B. Herrick of Chicago published a study in the *Journal of the American Medical Association* that concluded that a heart attack—a myocardial infarction, or death of heart muscle—didn't have to be fatal. It was a direct contradiction of the era's sclerotic dogma (heart attack = death), and it would eventually change most of the accepted thinking about cardiovascular disease. The study was a follow-up to a 1912 Herrick paper in *JAMA* that had met with near-universal indifference, a reaction that had stunned the doctor. But his 1919 publication had the advantage of an electrocardiograph machine to measure the heart's electrical impulses. The implications were enormous, even if they took even more years to be appreciated. In time, they would reveal the cardio epidemic.

Mom remembers almost nothing about that day, Saturday, February 2, 1963, when the epidemic found Dad for the first time as he was tapping on a ceiling tile in the basement on Wilshire Drive. She remembers only that earlier in the day she had attended a fund-raising luncheon of the local York chapter of the American Heart Association (true story) and then came home to a husband in acute distress. Her subsequent memory is of our being assembled in the early evening at the Flicks, York Crowd family friends, to catch our breath and contemplate the new reality. That's it. Nor is she interested in remembering more.

I was at basketball practice—St. Joe's Black Knights fifth-sixth–grade team—across town in West York, at the old York Catholic High School building. Mr. Grady gave me a ride home. Our house on Wilshire Drive was dark, empty, foreboding, though I admit that's hindsight talking. Then suddenly Mr. Grady was back in the driveway, suggesting that I come to his place. After some time there, Mr. Flick arrived to take me to his house. On that ride, more hindsight: why had *he* picked me up? At Flicks I walked into a crowded kitchen. Mom and Kathy, Mr. and Mrs. Flick, Jeff, Linda, Steve, Barbie, Greg, and Amy. I'd bet Mr. and Mrs. Philbin were there, more York Crowd friends; Mr. and Mrs. Ochs and Judy Ochs, too, Kathy's best friend, from across the street. Everyone there, gathered. I looked for Mom. There she was—thin lips, square jaw. Now I knew: something was wrong. Mom and Dad were supposed to go out tonight for Mrs. Schmitt's birthday. Mom took me to the downstairs powder room. I can still see the pink toilet and sink, the knit cover on the extra roll of toilet paper sitting on the tank. *Dad's in the hospital. He'll be okay. He had a heart attack.*

Did Mom drive Dad to the hospital or call for an ambulance from Springettsbury Township? Did she go to the emergency room, or was Dad admitted directly through his family doctor? Mom won't say and there are no records extant. In today's world, the chances are about 50-50 that Mom drove Dad to the hospital, because that's how about half the people in an "emergent cardiac situation" get there. Someone drives them. Or sometimes they drive themselves. Not a good idea. "Time is muscle," as the saying goes in heart attack circles. The longer it takes to get to treatment, the more muscle dies. And it's not coming back.

When Dad got to the hospital emergency room, he received the hospital's state-of-the-art care, circa the Kennedy Administration. He was probably hooked up to a six-lead electrocardiogram to gather some rudimentary information. He was likely administered Coumadin as an anticoagulant. If the pain was severe there would have been morphine. He was placed on oxygen. Time, however, was not of the essence. In 1963, York Hospital was still five years from its first heart catheterization. Dad's personal physician would have been called, and once he arrived, however long it took, he was in charge. That is not as awful as it may sound to our ears today. Just seeing his own doctor walk into the emergency room could have proved a major tonic for Dad. Dad's doctor knew Dad, a huge plus. He applied this knowledge, listened with his stethoscope, observed his patient. He then found Dad a bed somewhere—anywhere—in the hospital. Once he got Dad to his room and flat on his back, he ordered him not to raise his arms above his head, a dictum in effect for weeks. He told Dad they had to rest his heart, assess the damage, give it a chance to come back—to find out if it could come back. Wait-and-see began.

State of the art, and we were grateful for it.

———

That first heart attack was in 1963. Six years later, after the heart attack that killed him, we buried Dad up in Buffalo because that's where Nana wanted him. This made perfect sense to me. Mom's every-summer treks to western New York had rendered the place familiar enough to me that taking him "back to Buffalo" seemed natural enough. Besides, Nana was clearly tickled with the funeral arrangements, which Mom had ceded to her. Only years later would I realize that Mom had her reasons, both practical and politic. When Dad's brother Tom died in 1960 (of acute pneumonia, the notice in the Buffalo paper said), Nana insisted that he be buried in Buffalo. Uncle Tom by then had been living in California for years. Dad flew out to accompany the body back. What Nana wanted, Nana got. It came as no real surprise, for instance, that when I was trying to ascertain why 231 Rodney had disappeared I also discovered that from 1922 forward the house had always been in Nana's name only.

I sat in Nana's parlor on Friday after we flew up to Buffalo and listened to her describe the cemetery, the site, all that, in animated fashion. It should have been the strangest conversation I had ever heard in my sixteen years, except it wasn't. Nana and I had once had another conversation, that one at York Hospital not long after Dad's first heart attack, and she had come down to visit. We were sitting downstairs, near the front door, waiting for Mom. Nana was sixty-nine by then. She looked at me grimly. "I have already buried a husband and two sons," she said. "I don't want to bury my final boy." She stood up to walk outside—"to get some air"—at which point a man coming in pushed hard on the door, slamming it right into her, a full, blind-sided body blow. It should have knocked her over, but Nana held her ground.

So now, six years later, we were in Buffalo to bury Nana's final boy. I listened as she described how great the view was from the grave, how she had gone ahead and purchased a second one right next to it for Mom. Everything about 231 Rodney had always smelled comfortable and permanent to me. Sitting there sunk into Nana's furniture, everything somehow still did. Dad had lived here when he was my age. We had come back to the right space.

=======

When Dad outgrew the quarry and its boyhood adventures, he turned his attentions—and later his storytelling—to serious hunting and fishing. By then the auburn-haired John had been permanently renamed "Red" by his buddies. (The inevitable "Magoo" thankfully having fallen by the wayside.) With Joe Folkman and Bob Murphy—"The Three Musketeers," Nana called them—they hunted for ring-necked pheasant out toward Clarence, east of Buffalo; rabbit north near Lockport; and partridge a good ways out, down on the Southern Tier, almost to Pennsylvania. They spent their Saturdays and Sundays in the fields, then drove back to the neighborhood, cleaned up, and headed to a rathskeller at Main and Fillmore for a meatball sandwich and a couple of beers. Murph was usually the one with the car. For a while it was a Hudson Terraplane, the Depression Era classic with flowing fenders, bug-eyed headlights, and elongated grille. A real beauty. Cost Murph $140 used, and he had to finance it. Once on the way back from a day of hunting one of the guys took off his boots and stuck his toes up into the heater under the dash and his socks caught fire, filling the car with feet-stinking, wool-burning smoke. Dad really laughed when he told that one.

He was a good man to hunt with, Dad was. I knew it even as a kid. He carried a Stevens double-barreled twelve-gauge shotgun from Savage Arms Corporation, and it came alive in his hands. He respected it, was perhaps even a little afraid of it. In the field Dad possessed an ever-present awareness of where his hunting partners were positioned. You could count on him, you could trust him. If he started on your left, he stayed on your left. And he'd be right there, straight across, not ahead, not behind. When hunting, details matter. The sport can be enjoyed only if pursued correctly, a value he instilled in me. I believe one of the reasons I stopped hunting as an adult was I could never trust anyone the way I could Dad.

"He knew how to work a field," Bob Murphy told me. "He knew where the birds would be." Even better, "he knew where they were likely to go." High praise for a hunter, from a hunter. Bob Murphy, eighty-eight years old, born two weeks after Dad, lived two streets down from Rodney, on Wakefield Avenue. He is also Uncle Bob, a prewar friend of Dad's long before he married Dad's sister Alice in 1948. He is not one given to easy chatter; hearing him confirm what I'd long thought of Dad the hunter filled me with the warmth of a sunny autumn day, crunching along behind him in a wake of dried leaves.

When the guys went hunting, Red was in charge. *We'll walk this hedgerow, Murph on the left. At the end, we'll pivot off Joe on the right, and come back along the tree line.* But most important, Uncle Bob said, "He didn't get lost." That was a critical skill, especially when going after partridge. When a pheasant flushes and you don't bring it down, it escapes in a loud squabble, then soars three fields over, mocking you all the way. Partridge get themselves quickly back to ground. So where partridge go, hunters go, paying no mind to trails and landmarks. But with Dad they never got lost. Follow Red's lead and they'd wind up back at the Terraplane, right where they'd left it.

I hunted and fished with Dad all the time. And one of the great dates on the McKee calendar was Opening Day for either one. They were surrounded with ritual, defined by them, the traditions first creating the anticipation, then intensifying it. On the Friday night before, Dad commandeered the dining room table—the only night he dared—throwing a pad over the delicate pine before spreading out his equipment to check it over, leaving time for a run to the sporting-goods store if needed. Hunting season came with the added element, quite literally, of the gun-cleaning agent Hoppe's Nitro Powder Solvent No. 9. A redolent, mysterious concoction, its aroma hung thick in the air, a sweet, oily fragrance. Yes, fragrance. Kathy says she always thought it was banana oil. My olfactory nerve remains hardwired to Hoppe's. It is such a powerful elixir I need only say the name and both its smell and that Friday night return to me in complete detail.

And then Saturday morning was Opening Day. It began officially at the York Diner around 8:30. Timing was important. "We'll let everybody else get out there at dawn," Dad would say. "Let them scare everything away, so when they get tired and leave at 7:30, everything will have moved back in by the time we get there." A ploy for more sleep, but I believed him anyway and appreciate it even more now. And so we'd linger at the York Diner. The original place was exactly that, an old-fashioned railcar at the dogleg corner of East Market, Haines Road, and, no lie, Memory Lane. In 1962, when the intersection was straightened, the diner disappeared. The establishment resurfaced down East Market, though now just another restaurant. But we still had the "Pancake Club." That's what he called it. We'd order a flapjack stack, three high, and eat them one carefully forked-out wedge at a time. No knife! There was an art to doing it right. Dad insisted. Only then could we head out.

One Opening Day fish story, with the added benefit of being true:

We were at Muddy Creek, south and east of York, out in the rolling farmlands. Muddy Creek was heavily stocked with trout every spring from a railroad car on the old Maryland & Pennsylvania line—the famed Ma & Pa—that ran parallel to its banks. Dad was a fly fisherman, but this early in April, with the water high and unmanageable, a foamy coffee-with-cream color, we fished worms. We worked our way downstream to a sandbar and a rock spit jutting into the water, the rapids around it swirling in giant pools, one on each side of the rock. And it was just the two of us, me and Dad, the Pancake Club having worked its magic on the rest of the Opening Day mob.

We found ourselves a couple of forked sticks, jammed them into the sand, pitched in our worms, set the rods on the sticks, and waited to catch "a cigarette fish." It galls me now to provide cigarettes a starring role here, but they deserve their billing. It took Dad about seven minutes to smoke a cigarette. He timed it. At Muddy Creek, in this favored spot, seven minutes was also about the time it took for our bait to travel counterclockwise through the entire pool, so long as it didn't get hung up on the branches and junk being pushed along by spring rains. Waiting for one cigarette to get smoked forced patience, especially on me. *You don't want to pull the worm out of the fish's mouth.* It also provided Dad the opportunity to smoke a cigarette, not that he needed one. Dad inhaled three packs a day, a sixty count. At seven minutes each, that's seven hours of smoking a day. Subtract seven hours for sleep, and Dad spent 40 percent of his life with a cigarette. When he stubbed out a butt, he'd go no more than ten minutes before lighting another nail, always cupping his hands around it and bending down some, whether the wind was blowing or not.

With Dad's cigarette monitoring my patience, his rod suddenly bent. At first we thought it was a snag. Then, with the action at the rod tip, we knew it was a fish. With a bit more movement, we knew it had size. But not until Dad had the landing net underneath it and it finally broke the surface could we see how much. A monster. Well, no. A brown trout, it would probably measure out at eighteen or nineteen inches, if he could land it. Good size for Muddy Creek—a certified Big One. Then it ran one last time. The line screamed off Dad's rod, and he answered back with a powerful line of oaths and epithets. He kept the rod high in his left hand, tip up, an even tension on the line. In his right hand he held the net, down low, ready for the scoop beneath. For a long second nothing happened, the only motion the quivering rod—trout and angler locked in the fisherman's pas de deux. So Dad did the only thing he could. He went in after it. When he emerged, soaked to the belt buckle, the fish in the net, still battling, Dad was whooping and hollering like I'd never heard him. Up on the bank, literally trembling with excitement, he sank to his knees. He held the fish with one hand and me by the shoulder with the other and shook me like a nickel carton of chocolate milk. I remember his green eyes darting and dancing as he continued to shout and yell, unable to form real words. Green eyes full of unrestrained joy, as happy as I ever saw them.

I have Dad's bamboo fly rod and I have his shotgun, but I don't fish and I don't hunt. I am not philosophically opposed to either. I just don't. After he died, a few of Dad's hunting buddies took me with them on a couple of their outings. Mr. Philbin, Mr. Masterson, Mr. Kirk, Mr. Leahy. I appreciated the effort then; I appreciate it now. But it was awkward and forced and it didn't work.

I have kept one other thing from those days hunting and fishing with Dad. Truth is, I don't remember him coming home with a fish, a pheasant all that often. It's probably why that day at Muddy Creek was so special because, in his own words, he got "skunked" plenty. So this is what I've kept: coming home with a fish or a pheasant wasn't the point. The being out there was. The doing, the trying. A single strike by a rising rainbow on a Mickey Finn could sustain Dad in the stream all day. He liked to use "wet" flies—expertly, effortlessly, endlessly wristing the streamer in a graceful arc into the the top end of a pool, then working it down the length of the water. Maybe the next cast . . . Out in the field hunting, I think what he enjoyed the most—I know I did—was the blood-pumping flurry when the pheasant went up, its brilliant plumage always a sight. A confounding cacophony of flapping wings and squawking voice box, and Dad would have only an instant to find it, see it, get a bead on it. For Dad it was all in that instant, everything in the balance, when he was as likely to fail as he was to succeed.

For a couple of years Dad had a hunting dog named Pirate. With or without the dog, though, when I was with him in the fields, before he got me my own 20-gauge and I could walk beside him, my job was to stay behind him as close as possible. When a bird went up I was to get to the ground immediately. One time when a pheasant flushed I ended up on my knees literally right next to him. The bird rose in a fury directly in front of us and then arched to our right and circled, gradually gaining distance. Dad, gun to his shoulder, followed the bird, slowly cork-screwing himself a full 360 degrees, swinging over me before finding his shot, by then the tail feathers nearly out of range. He pulled the triggers on both barrels simultaneously. The explosions filled my ears with thunder and my nose with gunpowder. I don't remember what happened next. And it doesn't matter.

———

What was Dad thinking when he had that first heart attack, while he was having that first heart attack? I often wonder. In 1963, a total of 546,813 people died of "arteriosclerotic heart disease, including coronary disease," according to the National Center for Health Statistics. Narrowing the search field, 26,116 people between the ages of forty and forty-nine succumbed. Of those, 18,726 were white men; 1,838 were black men. But somehow, for some reason, Dad had not added his number to that ledger. It is difficult even to know how truly severe his heart attack was, given the times. How bad could it have been if it didn't kill him? Of course, what did he know then? And what do I know now? He was in the basement. He came upstairs. He took some Tums. He stretched out in bed. What went through his mind when he finally understood this wasn't "indigestion"?

Richard Pryor, in his 1979 concert film, tells the story of his own heart attack. He digs his fist into his chest and throws himself to the stage. Within seconds he is on his back begging not to die, pleading with his heart not to kill him. Was it like that for Dad? I want to know, but I can't. So I have asked others to tell me, piecing their stories together into a single tale.

Four or five months before the heart attack, I'm raking pine needles in my yard. I remember a sensation coming over me. I can describe it this way: perhaps you've ridden down a road, a tree-lined road on a sunny day, and the sun is going in and out of the trees as you're driving and that gives you a momentary sense of, not lightheadedness, but a disorientation. I had that. This happened twice before the heart attack. Both times I was raking pine needles.

It got so I was not able to walk up a half a flight of steps. I was walking from the parking lot into the hospital [speaker is a physician]; I was walking a little slower so I wouldn't get any symptoms. I tried to ignore it. But it got to where I couldn't. The capacity for people to ignore is real big.

Whatever this is, I can shake it off, I can take care of it. That whole river-in-Egypt thing. Denial, yeah, it was there.

The only warning I had—and this is only looking back— was two days [before], I have a stationary bike in the basement and that's what I was doing that weekend. And on Saturday I couldn't finish my routine. And I thought, "That's really strange. I must be tireder than I thought."

I'm thinking, "I'm in better shape than this." But then it's, "I'm in worse shape than I thought." Or I got the flu or something. But no, the words "heart attack" never crossed my mind until I walked into the house and I saw the look on my wife's face.

I rowed the morning of my heart attack. November sixteenth. I left the boathouse, and I remember standing on the steps and feeling this bead of sweat coming off my forehead, just one bead rolling over my left eye. I'd just showered and I'm saying, "Geez, it's chilly. That shouldn't be happening."

I was exercising and I couldn't finish my routine. I had to sit down. I made it up the stairs and sat down in the kitchen, and my wife took one look at me and said, "We're going to the emergency room."

Fever and aches and pains and eventually the runs. And it was extreme. At about 5:30 in the morning I got a call to the bathroom. As soon as I got there, I had what I can only describe as a wavelike sensation that came over me. A profound lightheadedness. It lasted about five seconds.

I was left with significant cold sweats and a bit of the shakes like when you've had that extra cup of coffee. And then the sensation in my chest. I'll describe it as pain, but that might be overstatement. It was hardly unendurable. It was just steady and THERE, right in the middle of my chest. Different from anything I'd ever felt before. Within seconds, within seconds, I knew I was having a heart attack. It was never in doubt, there was never a question about it. I knew.

I lay down on the front walk in front of our house. And then nobody drove by for probably thirty minutes. I called my husband, but I didn't realize the call hadn't gone through. Then I just kind of waited. I actually cried out for help for a little while, but nobody heard me. Then I got tired and was terrified. I knew something was really wrong with me, and I just wanted the ambulance to get there. So I called my husband again, and I just kind of said, "Help. Please help me."

I never had any real pain. I never had significant discomfort. Everything I had was subtle. This tiny, tiny, barely discernible sensation, a pain in my chest. I'd heard of the giant pains. But this was so subtle, you know?

I took the kids ice skating at a local pond. They get going and I'm putting my skates on and all of a sudden I am huffing and puffing. I just felt totally, absolutely weak. I get everybody out of their skates and get all the kids into

*the van up the hill and start driving back to the house. I
don't know I'm having a heart attack, right? So now I'm
driving and I'm fading in and out. My older daughter is
in the front. She's making sure I stay awake. "Here comes
a turn, Dad." Or, "Slow down, Dad, here's a stop sign."
Trying to drive home was dumb. It was a huge chance to
take with three kids in the car. But I don't know what else
I could have done. This was twelve years ago. We didn't
have cellphones. I pull into the driveway and just kind of
stagger into the house, the kids yelling at Mom to call
nine-one-one.*

*I was in my car and I began to sweat, started to feel kind
of clammy. [Four miles later] I'm starting to feel nause-
ated. [Then], as I was getting onto the expressway, I kind
of felt there was something going on. I recall thinking
that I need to get to the shoulder because I didn't want to
take anybody out with me. I remember looking in the
rearview mirror and checking myself out and realizing
how gray my face looked.*

*I had pain in my chest and in my left arm. And I knew
immediately what it was. I [later] asked my wife, "Exactly what did I say to you?" And she said, "Well, you
just very calmly said, 'I'm having a heart attack.' And
that was it."*

*It was like this total global body kind of thing. I felt so
weird.*

I lost power. I was just totally drained. [I'm a rower], and I know how much it takes for me to move around. I know what power is. [And then] not to have any power at all . . .

I'm sitting in the car [on the shoulder]. I call nine-one-one. . . . Then my foreman from work calls to tell me that he wasn't going to be in next Thursday, or something. And I said, "I'm not sure I'm going to be around next Thursday. I got something going on here. I can't tell exactly what it is, but there's something serious going on here."

I had a cold. The [paramedics] got there and they kind of pronounce, well, you should probably go to the emergency room and have this cold checked out. They're packing up and getting ready to go out the door. I don't remember this, but my wife tells me that my eyes rolled back into my head, and now it was clear what was going on. The EMS guys paddled me right there and rushed me to the hospital.

I never thought of anything other than call the ambulance and get to the hospital. And that's not in character. I'd virtually never been to a hospital. Like lots of people, I avoid, I procrastinate. But in that minute there was no other thought than "Get me to the hospital!"

The phone dropped into my lap. A period of time went by. I don't know how long. It could have been ten minutes, twenty, thirty. But it seemed like a good time to call nine-one-one back. I said, "I'm dying out here. I'm in bad shape."

I had some indigestion but didn't think much of it. Later I'm watching television and I start getting this stinging sensation in my arm. My wife went to bed and then I followed. I'm laying down for maybe forty-five minutes when my chest starts to pound. I sit up and say, "I'm having a heart attack. You better call nine-one-one." I put my pants on and walked down the steps into the dining room. But I couldn't go any farther. I put myself down. I knew there was something wrong and I didn't want to get into any more trouble, so I just put myself on the floor.

My principal emotion was one of anger, not fear and not a deep concern, but anger. I remember saying to my wife in very profane terms: "Can you believe this? I am going to die right here on the freaking living room floor. I'm going to die right here, can you believe it?"

The fire station is just a couple of blocks away. I'm lying on the floor, and I can hear the sirens. They were here in no time at all.

We're in rush-hour traffic. I tried to do deep breathing to try to calm myself down. I tried to concentrate on where we were going. You know, try to figure out the route they were taking just to keep my mind on something else. But I was really scared. I knew there was something really wrong with me. I just prayed, "Get me to the hospital where they can do something."

I'm in the ambulance . . . and I say to one of the guys working on me, "I guess I can figure that I'm having a heart attack, right?" And he said, "We're not allowed to tell you." So, okay, in this day and age, "I can't tell you" means, "You're having a heart attack." And then just a couple of minutes later I hear on one of their radios, "We have a guy in his early fifties having a massive, massive heart attack!"

It just hurt so bad. I was just laying there and there was just so much pressure on my chest—coming straight down on my chest.

I felt like my whole body, it practically felt like it was shuddering. Everything felt like it was seizing inside me. It was a violent feeling. It was uncomfortable but not painful. It almost felt like I was going to have this huge bowel movement or something. I felt this tremendous pounding inside me, like something was violently moving around.

I never thought I was having a heart attack. It was just, "What the hell's going on here?"

I had a calm in this experience that I cannot explain to you in any objective terms. It was really quite amazing. There was never a fear of dying. Rationally, I knew it was a possibility, but there was never a fear of it. I don't think

I really thought that I was going to die. I guess that's maybe it.

It feels like there's an elephant sitting on my chest. The classic. But there was just so much pressure. It's on your heart, but it's pounding in your head.

The pounding was just too much. I just kept saying, "Stay calm. Stay calm." But the pain was just always there. It was constant.

I thought about a lot of things. I thought about my wife. I thought about my kids. I thought about what I've done with my life. But I didn't think about any of that for long, because all I could really think about was the pain.

All that mortality stuff, it looms. That whole, will-I-be-here-tomorrow thing, it does go through your mind. You pray: I hope I'm okay, because I'm not done here.

I was on the table [in the emergency room], and I had to throw up. When I did, I felt everything rush out of me. I felt better, but that's exactly how it felt to me, that everything had rushed out of me. All the pressure was gone, and it felt like it was gone, but that scared the shit out of me. It was very scary. Everything had been pounding for such a long time and hurting. And then everything rushed out, and I felt like I was dropping out of it. That was the scariest point. I felt like I was going.

It was just a snap of a finger. It was that fast. But I felt like I was going.

I remember thinking that this could be an all-or-nothing situation. But I wasn't afraid. Because, well, here it is. Whatever happens, happens. That's the way it is. I don't know if it was a helplessness or just surrendering to the fates. I remember being more disappointed than the whole mortality thing. That I wasn't going to be here; I wouldn't be around for my daughter's graduation.

They wanted someone to stay with me that first night in the ICU because they were afraid I was going to try to get up. I was loony. My mom volunteered. And it was only when she and I were alone, just briefly, that it kind of finally sunk in that something had happened. And I cried for probably three minutes. "Mom, why did this have to happen to me?" You know?

I don't think I ever went into as deep a funk [after the attack]. But I do remember one specific afternoon. My wife was home with the kids. I was sitting in bed looking out the window and having the deepest feeling of, you know, life really sucks. Why did this happen to me? I'm only forty-something years old. GODDAMNIT!

———

Dad stayed flat on his back in York Hospital for a month, resting his heart. And the doctor meant it when he told Dad he couldn't raise his arms above his head. He spent nearly two more months at home. At this point the doctor told Dad to start getting some exercise, in the form of slow walking that gingerly extended into something longer. Only then did Dad take his first steps back to Cole Steel and the warehouse and all those desks and office chairs and file cabinets that had to be moved through the place with all due haste. And every day for the rest of his life Dad came home for lunch and a short nap.

Those hospital days were a time out of time. We settled into a new routine. Mom got us off to school, then headed to the "horse-pistol." That's what we called it, an unreal word for an unreal place. She would be back on Wilshire Drive by the time we got home, unless she picked us up after school to go visit Dad. I loved going to the hospital. Seeing Dad was great and all, but that wasn't it. You had to be twelve years old to visit. I was ten. But like every year of my life except for eighth grade, I was big for my age, the tallest in my class. Dad had his heart attack on Groundhog Day; on February 3, I became two years older. This drips with symbolism, but I hadn't a clue. I just reveled in Mom's order to act older, stand straighter.

There were victories. One stands above the rest. Two, maybe three weeks in, Mom's sister Ev came down for a visit. Her son Tommy drove her. He is almost ten years older than I am. That's a huge gap when you're the much-younger cousin, and he was always a mystery to me. He came along expressly to shave Dad, give him a haircut, clean him up. Dad was meticulous in his grooming—not vain, just precise. He shaved every day even when we were on vacation, camping somewhere from Maine to Tennessee to Canada. There he'd be, circular mirror hanging from a tree branch, hot water steaming in a plastic basin, cleaning himself up for another day of fishing, fire building, and popcorn making. Once on one of our trips to Maine's Acadia National Park, Kathy talked him into not shaving, to growing a beard, to *being cool*. Dad obliged, for the entire two weeks, and it damn near killed him.

To be flat on your back in a hospital bed unable to raise your arms, that's debilitating enough. To lie there with nothing to do but think about your beard getting longer and your hair not getting combed—well, I can feel Dad's anxiety down into my fingertips even as I type this. Then Tommy came and saved the day. I mean that. It remains stunning to realize what a huge deal this was. Shave and a haircut, that's it. I see Tommy leaning over, working on Dad, their noses close. I hear the blade rasping against his skin. I feel how good it must have made Dad feel, arms at his side, as his face and his self were slowly restored, razor stroke by razor stroke.

THURSDAY, OCTOBER 2

She came early and left quickly. I see her standing in front of Dad's casket, alone in the room save for Mom next to her not knowing quite what to do. Her hair was swirled in a beehive. Her glasses, big dark things with rhinestone wings, dominated her face. She stood there looking at Dad, daubing at her reddened nose with a tissue, crying, crying, crying.

It was too early in the night for a receiving line (though Mom had meticulously prepped both me and Kathy on our expected roles), so I sat in a chair against a far wall, taking in one more weirdness of what had already been two very weird days. Everything had turned so strange that nothing seemed strange at all.

Her name was . . . does it matter? It's that I still remember it. She told Mom she had worked for Dad at Cole Steel. Though she wasn't Dad's secretary, his "Gal Friday," as such indispensable women were then known. We knew Dad's secretary. She hovered on the edge of our family, a real, valued presence. She was important to Dad, ergo, important to us.

No, this woman crying next to Mom had worked for Dad, perhaps in the general secretarial pool, perhaps in another department that had regular dealings with Dad's warehouse. Actually, I have no idea. All I know is she came to the Keffer Funeral Home on Mount Rose Avenue early that night, cried inconsolably, was comforted by Mom, and left before the viewing proper started.

So, a question. Was this Dad's girlfriend? I might have asked myself that while sitting there watching it all unfold, though probably not in so many words. I also dismissed it out of hand, if only because I had too many other things going on to grapple with that, too. It would be years before I asked again. I was in my thirties at least, maybe my forties. Eventually, I asked Kathy. More eventually, I even asked Mom.

Was she? In a word, no. Of all three of us, asked and answered. We could be completely wrong, of course. I am way past the point when one finally realizes that anything—*anything*—is possible. Still, I say no.

Here's the thing. I am now also old enough to understand how a guy who cheats on his wife would have to act so he could cheat on his wife. And then how he'd behave once he did. Dad didn't, on either count. He was never not home. And when he wasn't home he was out at the farm trying to fix something or out in the fields or the creeks hunting and fishing. I know this because I was with him. He came home from work every night at 6:15 P.M. You could set your clock on it. Quitting time was 5:00, but Dad, ever the captain, insisted on being the last off the ship. He rarely left before 5:30. That got him home during *The Huntley-Brinkley Report* on WGAL-TV Channel 8, the NBC affiliate out of Lancaster, Pennsylvania, the only station our huge black-and-white television set regularly picked up. (On occasion we could get a snowy image from Philadelphia; it might as well have been from Mars.)

Dad would open the door and whistle. He was a terrific whistler, perfect pitch, sweet sound. You enjoyed it because he enjoyed it. His home-from-work greeting was just two notes, the first beat twice as long as the second, a quick rise and a fall: *DOOT-doot*. I am sure he let loose with it when he got home that last Tuesday night. We'd hear his whistle and know Dad was home and all was where it was supposed to be, again. As a very little kid—when a father's nightly return still possesses its routine magic—I'd run to him and kiss him on the cheek, his stubble bristling my lips. On winter days his skin would be cold, but just on the surface. I knew there was warmth beneath.

He loathed the business trips, did everything he could to get out of them. He whined before, complained after. He winnowed these commitments to one or two a year, at most, quick out-and-backs. In doing so, by accident or design he transformed them into huge dates on the McKee calendar— complete aberrations, total discombobulations, full of gifts upon his return.

Also, he was enough of a Catholic that his religion wouldn't have allowed it. I believe that. I never saw Dad as a spiritual sort, but I think Catholicism was important to him. He had spent his high school years plus an additional year at the minor seminary. He had endured them at his mother's insistence, but they had had their effect. He had been an altar boy, too, another source of his stories, about getting himself out of bed, on his own, and trudging to Blessed Trinity four blocks from Rodney, on a cold Buffalo morning with the snow coming off Lake Erie, to serve the 6:30 Mass. They were depending on him. Once, when I was a boy, he came home from a morning Mass at St. Joe's in York (likely getting a Holy Day of Obligation out of the way early) to announce delightedly that the priest had rung the entrance bell himself and come out solo, so Dad had walked up to the Communion rail, unhooked the maroon sash, rehooked it behind him, and served as altar boy. Entering the sanctuary of a Catholic Church, especially then, was an act not done lightly. He was just tickled about it, remembering when to switch the book from one side of the altar to the other, how to pour the wine into the chalice at the Offertory, when to ring the bell during the Consecration—all the little details that had become a part of him thirty, thirty-five years before.

Finally, this. We were still on Wilshire Drive, so I was no more than eight, nine years old. Dad had a business dinner to which he was required to take his secretary, some sort of appreciation banquet, no spouses allowed. When a fumbling Dad explained it to Mom, even I could tell it was a bizarre dynamic. To add to the weirdness, the bosses were expected to pick up their secretaries and drive them to the event, like on an actual date or something. It was as if a couple of bosses who *were* doing their female underlings had planned the whole thing to have one night of not slinking around. From today's vantage, it is impossible to imagine such an event even taking place. Dad clearly, certainly wished it wasn't about to then. Same for Mom. She did not cotton to her role in their Helen-

and-Red partnership being so casually dismissed. When Dad came home beforehand to change, he was in a strange, unsettled mood, fully incapable of masking how he felt.

If I protest too much, so be it. And I realize any argument for can be used against. But here's one final reason I believe what I believe. Mom and Dad really loved each other.

When you ask Mom a question about her side of the family—one of time: when so-and-so was born, when such-and-such happened—her response is so predictable it has become its own parody. "Well, let's see," she'll say, "Marg and Leo were married in 1940 . . ." and she works forward from there. Marg is Mom's older sister by nine years, and her conveniently round-numbered wedding date has become Mom's B.C./A.D. touchstone. That date—July 20—is also the day when Dad first met Mom's family. I should say "was supposed to meet" Mom's family. A year later Mom would meet Jack and Anna McKee, and Jack would die of a heart attack driving back from the lake. Dad had his problems, too, when meeting Mom's family. Thankfully, no one died; Dad just got himself thrown in jail.

The plan was for Dad to pick up Mom, one of the maids of honor at Marg's wedding, back at Frank and Margaret Reedy's summer cottage on what was then Maple Street in Angola-By-The-Lake after the reception. Aunt Margaret Reedy was Mom's mother's sister. I see it like this: Mom, still in her wedding finery, a flowered gown with sash, peering through a window down Maple Street, anxiously awaiting Dad's arrival. Eight P.M., the appointed time, no Red McKee. Nine P.M., ten

P.M., eleven P.M. She finally gives up, embarrassed, and goes disconsolately to bed.

Next morning, first thing, here comes Red McKee, driving up in his dad's car, sheepish look on his face. Meet now Uncle Frank. I never did, but through Mom's sister Ev, the designated O'Neil storyteller who knew well not to let the facts stand in the way of a good story, I came to know him as a larger-than-life, white-haired Irishman whose bellowing voice could fill the room, and then some. He engendered absolute love or total terror, often simultaneously. "He was quick to defend if he thought someone had dared slight his family," Mom confirms. How dare this East Buffalo kid stand up his niece!

Apparently, though, Uncle Frank allowed Dad to state his case. The brakes on his dad's car were shot. Coming down the Lake Shore Road from Buffalo, he'd made a left onto Beach Road, about a mile from Maple. The brakes failed and the car went off to the right, into a row of rental bikes at a house owned by a woman named Maisie. She called the cops and had Dad thrown in jail overnight, no questions, no phone call. With this, according to Aunt Evie's telling, Uncle Frank had heard enough and exploded. But not at Dad—at Maisie the Bike Lady. *How dare she! This fine young man seeing my niece! I should have* her *arrested!* I picture Dad in the Reedy's front room, ears pinned to the wall by Uncle Frank's force of nature, absolutely no clue what he has just walked into, no idea what to say, what to do. What he couldn't have known was that Uncle Frank had already brought him inside the O'Neil castle. For years, Mom says, "all you had to do to get Uncle Frank going was say, 'Maisie the Bike Lady.'"

That was 1940, round-numbered, convenient. Mom and Dad wouldn't be married for another seven years. Much history was still to happen, most of the story not of their writing. Dad would need most every day of it. If he had quickly won over Uncle Frank, it would take much longer to win his niece. There were the boyfriends, for one thing. There was also her obvious independent streak. So obvious it must have been some of what appealed so much to Dad.

In July 1942, with Dad not yet in the service, Mom quit her secretarial job at H.I. Sackett Electric to take off with her best friend from across the street (and friend for life), Aggie Mahoney, on a long-planned bus trip to Mexico. Her boss's son was "a body grabber," Mom says, and she was looking for an excuse to get out, her only option. Besides, the war was on, and she knew she could get a better job when she got back—which she did, at Bell Aircraft, making $40 a week, nearly twice her Sackett wage and at half the aggravation. It was a better job, too: "Men were scarce. I got to do a lot of the stuff that they would have done."

Mom's Mexico sojourn has assumed legendary status within our family. One, because for years Mom told Kathy and me that she and Aggie made the trip in a prewar 1941. Taking that trip the next year, the world at war, might seem frivolous and selfish. But together they had been saving their nickels for a couple of years; no way they weren't going. Two, the mere fact that they did it. Mom, twenty-one; Aggie, twenty-three; two girls off on their own when girls weren't off on their own.

We have a picture of Mom in Acapulco. Just a snapshot quickly shuttered, but it captured her in near-perfect, pensive profile, thumb of her left hand under her chin, manicured nails dark and polished. In her right hand is a cigarette. Her hair, pulled back off her face, cascades past her shoulders onto a sweater, striped and shapely. No wonder all the boyfriends; no wonder Dad's determination. In 1978, Noreen and I backpacked Europe, and we caught up to Mom and Aggie on another of their trips, this one to the Costa del Sol in Spain. Aggie—funny, smart, agnostic, yin to mom's yang—regaled us with stories of that Mexico trip, most of them about a leggy 5-foot-8-inch Helen O'Neil and her golden-red hair and how she turned heads everywhere they went. (Many years after that Spain trip, Mom protested that Aggie had poured too much blarney that night. Yes, in Mexico Mom did wear the one bikini of her life, or what passed for one back then, and she did catch the fancy of a guy named Adrian, but Aggie meanwhile was dating Jorge—*a general in the Mexican Air Force.* "We gave them up," Mom said. "They were too fast for us!" And there were no more gentleman adventures for the rest of the trip.)

Once Mom got back to Buffalo and Bell Aircraft—*DUH Bells*, as it was called—Dad might have claimed his bride. It was Mom, in fact, who broached the subject of marriage before Dad went into the service in 1943. At least three of her friends had already walked the aisle, and there was pressure on all young women to do the same. Looking back, Mom says, she probably got caught up in the romance of the time. It was the least she could do for a man off to war, that sort of thing. But Dad—practical Dad and dutiful son—said no. If they were married, Mom, not Nana, would receive the government benefits should the worst befall him. "Your father was more sensible about things like that," Mom says. And in fact there would be a government benefit. Dad fell on his rifle during training and it rather grotesquely pierced him in the groin, resulting in a long varicose vein running down the inside of his leg. Nana received a check until she died—for years it was $17 a month.

A married Mrs. John McKee, Jr., might also have moved in with Nana at 231 and assumed the role of the waiting wife back home, all of which seems merely impossible in hindsight. By January 1945, Mom was working in Washington, D.C., a secretary in the War Department, in the Civilian Personnel Branch of the Chief of Engineers. (Her goal once upon a time to go to college had also included "someplace not in Buffalo.") She and Aggie were in a taxi on Pennsylvania Avenue in front of the White House on April 12 when they heard on the radio that President Roosevelt (suffering from high blood pressure and severe heart disease, in addition to polio) had died of a cerebral hemorrhage in Warm Springs, Georgia. Later that year Mom noticed on a bulletin board that Robert Jackson, the U.S. Supreme Court justice, was assembling a staff for Germany, where he was to serve as the lead American prosecutor at the coming Nuremberg War Crimes Trial. Mom may have had a sense of history, but more immediately she had a need for money. She had recently totaled her dad's car. The secretarial job at "Headquarters, European Theater of Operations, Nuremberg" would, with the 25 percent overseas differential, bump her up to $2,900 a year. She arrived in October 1945 on an air transport, about a month before the trials began.

If we hold Mom's Mexico trip in high esteem, her nearly seven months in Nuremberg are merely off the chart. That her duties precluded her from attending the proceedings themselves doesn't matter. *My mother was at the Nuremberg Trials!* How many times did I blurt that out during a history class? And Mom says that she at times did attend, getting a pass from her boss "when something big was going to happen." That puts her in the second-floor courtroom of the Palace of Justice in mid-March 1946, the corpulent Hermann Göring, Hitler's successor to the Third Reich, in the witness stand. I asked Mom what she remembers. "Well, he wasn't thin," she said. I wondered if she had an awareness that she was in the presence of a great evil, its very personification. No, she said, actually not. What she remembers is being aware of how absolutely charming he was. Or, rather, how absolutely charming he thought he was. And she couldn't understand why people hadn't realized that he wasn't.

The gravity of the trials notwithstanding (or perhaps for that reason), in southern Germany Mom quite simply "had a ball." She was twenty-five, far from home, on her own. There were side trips to Prague, Czechoslovakia. Another to St. Moritz, Switzerland, where she skied the Alps and rode the bobsleigh run that in two more years would be the Olympic course. In Paris, in the restaurant on the second level of the Eiffel Tower, she bumped into a serviceman she knew from Buffalo. Actually, he was a good friend of the man with the three-part German name. He was thrilled beyond measure to see a girl from home. "We danced all night," Mom says. Also in Nuremberg there was the one final beau before Dad, one final road not taken. He was a captain in the Army Air Corps, a lawyer on Jackson's staff, seven years her senior, and he was at least as dashing, to hear Mom tell, as it all might suggest. They flew over together on the transport, would return together on the SS *Westerly Victory*, leaving, in the parlance of the time, "Le Havre 23 April, arriving New York 2 May." She had become the leading lady in her own black-and-white postwar matinee romance.

Meanwhile, back in Buffalo, Dad came home from the war and the South Pacific the first week of January 1946, then had to wait for Mom to get back from Germany. Surely not the way he'd planned it. When Mom returned, in short order she went to New Jersey to meet the parents of her Air Corps captain. She scored significant points with his mother, an Italian immigrant, when her son took Mom to church on Sunday, even if he did wait in the car. And a brother remarked to Mom that the captain sure seemed in an "expansive mood" with her around. But at the bus station with Mom heading back, he pecked her on the cheek and said something like, "I'll call ya, kid." And that was that. She never heard from him again.

Once more in Buffalo, again she wasted little time, moving to New York City in June. She never made it to college, but by now she obviously had an exact sense of her own worth. She took a job with Morrison-Knudsen Afghanistan, a foreign construction company. She lived with Aggie in Brooklyn Heights across the East River from Manhattan. Dad followed, determined. If he had made the right decision back in 1942, he was not going to make the wrong one now. He took a railroad flat on Second Avenue in the city, bathtub in the kitchen, bathroom down the hall. It was late summer 1946. They had known each other for eight years; spent most of the last four apart. They had seen the world, lived its story from the inside. They married on November 8, 1947, at St. John the Evangelist Church on Seneca Street, two blocks from Seneca Parkside, on a snowy weekend up from New York. Mom was nearly twenty-seven, Dad almost twenty-nine. Only now does it seem as certain as the water that thunders over Niagara Falls, where they honeymooned. The priest was Father Anthony McKee, Dad's cousin. Mom wore a dark-green velvet full-length suit with a wide matching hat, an ensemble that would have done Scarlett O'Hara proud.

———

The woman with the beehive hair and winged glasses? I have been asking the wrong question. The right question, the salient question is this: Was Dad good at his job?

By "good," I don't mean "successful." By any objective measure of the times he was, in a modest, middle-class sort of way, which was all he had ever wanted. House in the 'burbs, a wife who worked though she didn't have to, two kids, two cars, two weeks' vacation, his own hunting dog, friends, standing in his church, the executive directorship of the Steel Office Furniture Association. For Christmas in 1966, Dad bought Mom a midnight-blue Oldsmobile Cutlass Supreme, a hard top with black-vinyl roof. A great-looking car, it was the first brand-new model that he bought up front and not at the end of the production year. And he wore a suit and tie and white shirt to the office every day. Not everybody's dad did. I was acutely aware of that, always understood the significance, at least obliquely. He was, after all, "the boss of the warehouse."

If I take this woman at face value, she came to the viewing to pay respects to a former boss who was worth crying over. Why? Because he was a good man to work for. I will always believe that Dad's job is part of what killed him—the boss, the stress, the deadlines. If he was just another S.O.B. in the corner office, then what was the point?

Dad did only one kind of work for most of his life: traffic management. I doubt, however, if initially it was a career choice. A kid from Rodney east of Main at the tail end of the Great Depression, a war on the way, wasn't thinking career. He was looking for a job. In 1938, the year after he left the seminary and the year he met Mom out at Sunset Bay, he was a truck driver and warehouse clerk for Ohio Chemical & Manufacturing, and he was probably damn grateful to have found the work. He delivered oxygen tanks to people's homes, wrestling 150-pound cylinders up stairs and into bedrooms. Knock off the valve and there could be trouble. There are stories of workers at Bethlehem Steel angling upturned cylinders, then snapping off the valve with a quick hit of a wrench to rocket them over Lake Erie.

There were other, similar jobs before the war. He was a dispatcher at A&B Fast Freight, and in his last job before he joined the service he was a traffic rate clerk for Curtiss-Wright, one of Buffalo's booming wartime airplane manufacturers. He also found employment at Trico Products Corporation, a maker of windshield wipers. Though you could say Trico found him. John R. Oishei, a theater manager, started the company in 1917 after his car had collided with a bicyclist on a rainy night. Mr. Oishei, who had barely seen the bicyclist (who wasn't hurt), saw opportunity. With local inventor John W. Jepson, Mr. Oishei marketed Jepson's "Rain Rubber," a handheld squeegee that the driver operated through a horizontal slit between upper and lower windshields. In not too many years "Tri-Continental Products Company" was supplying most of Detroit with the latest in wiper technology.

Dad got the job because he used to fish sometimes in Delaware Park, where he befriended a fellow angler—and a brother of Mr. Oishei. It is not difficult to picture. Dad possessed an easy manner, particularly with a fishing rod in his hands. *Any luck? What bait you usin'? Try this one.* Whether this Oishei directed Dad to the Trico traffic department or that's where the opening was isn't known. But Dad's duties included routing Trico trucks through the city so as to keep the various-heighted vehicles from smacking into bridges and electric wires. Aunt Alice recalls Dad being excited not just by the work but also by the responsibility. It was while at Trico in 1940 and 1941 that Dad netted himself a career as sure as he would the big one at Muddy Creek years later.

Then came December 7, 1941. Dad and his pal Bob Murphy from two streets down on Wakefield were hunting rabbit up in Lockport north of the city that Sunday. There was no snow on the ground, which was different, Uncle Bob remembers. Then everything became different. Early in the afternoon they searched out a cafe and left Sally, Dad's beagle, in the car. It was always chili for lunch when out on the hunt.

They walked in knowing nothing. Inside, the radio was on and the people told them everything.

At his widowed mother's request, Dad, the dutiful son, filed for hardships and remained in Buffalo. He wasn't inducted for another year; he left for basic training the first week of 1943. He was mustered out on New Year's Day 1946, and he came home with the Asiatic-Pacific Medal and the Philippines Liberation Ribbon. I'm guessing the Air Corps gave out lots of those. Dad was a quartermaster, a noncommissioned officer whose civilian work experience got put to at least some good use in the military. He built and maintained gas depots; later, he kept supplies coming to the commissaries. And he was in some demand to build showers with hot water. He shipped out for the South Pacific in November 1943 and carried out his orders well behind the front lines, with only an occasional foray anywhere near the perimeter. Three miles of New Guinea jungle, he wrote home, was keeping him far from "Tojo." He had enough free time to take correspondence courses from the University of Tennessee traffic-management school. He and a couple of buddies for a while had a pet pig named "Bosco." The snapshots we have of him from that time are fun-loving, carefree, even innocent. A couple show how the war came to him, not he to it. In one he is standing next to an airplane. Painted on the fuselage in quite exact detail is a scantily clad woman with long, luxurious hair. Rita Hayworth, perhaps. There is Dad, skinny and leather-faced, squinting into the sun, left arm akimbo, right hand planted firmly on a very ample left breast. "Hands Astray" is inked along the picture's edge in nervous printing.

The closest Dad got to the front was in a story he liked to tell on himself, of the one time his unit was warned of a possible Japanese attack. Dad went to bed with his rifle. In the middle of the night someone grabbed his shoulder and shook him. They were here! That's when he shot up, wide awake. His own hand had grabbed his own shoulder. And that's when he would start laughing about how he damn near scared himself to death in defense of his country.

But as it must have been for countless men of his generation, I think World War II was for Dad the defining moment, the one from which there was no return. Dad saw none of the war's horrors, but he was one of the many, many American servicemen who never stopped believing that without the atom bombs dropped on Hiroshima and Nagasaki he wouldn't be alive, because he was slated for the invasion of Japan. I can hear him saying it, in those words. As it was, it never came to that, making Dad's war something akin to the old-fashioned world tour that the Newport scions once embarked upon. It took him all over the South Pacific and Australia and for a time to Japan during the early months of the occupation. It was involuntary and soaked in a homesickness relieved only by the next letter from home, but that didn't make it any less the grand adventure, any less farther from Buffalo, and all a kid from the quarry had ever known.

He would occasionally burst out laughing, for no apparent reason. He could be watching TV, driving, anything. He'd suddenly start laughing, a laugh of obvious delight that he would try to stifle but never quite could. Trying to quell it only made him guffaw the more. He'd get going, and we knew he was somewhere back . . . there. Sometimes he tried to get us in on the joke, but that rarely succeeded. We learned to let him go, to let him laugh until it left him.

I have long been intrigued by this exact moment in Dad's life, when he returned from the South Pacific. In 1976—I was about the same age he had been in that postwar era—I returned to Buffalo and Rodney Avenue for the first time since he had died. I went to talk to Nana and Aunt Mary Jane about Dad, to hear specifically what he had been like when he got back home. I sat in the upstairs kitchen with Aunt Mary Jane in the only house she had ever lived in, where she had raised six children. The neighborhood had become something very different from what it had once been. But not here in this house, not in this kitchen.

Mom says that Aunt Mary Jane and Dad could have been twins, they were that much alike. Aunt Mary Jane loved to laugh. Her giggle was toothy and infectious. But when I asked her about Dad after the war, she turned wistful. Everything was different when he got back, she said, about Buffalo, about him. He couldn't sit still. Literally. He was twenty-seven. He wanted to get to the rest of his life. This turn of events was particularly difficult on her and Alice. Once upon a time 231 Rodney had been the neighborhood place for Dad and his buddies. A testament to Dad perhaps (he was in charge on the hunt, after all) but also to the fact that Red McKee had a pair of kid sisters, redheads both. And Nana made a great shrimp salad. Mary Jane hoped it would be what it used to be when he got back, she said, with Dad and the guys sitting around the kitchen table with a couple of Genesee beers, goofing on "Janie" and "A."

But there was no time for that after the war. In 1937, about when an eighteen-year-old Dad had first entered the job market, the federal government had just bailed out Buffalo. Then came war. Buffalo, perfectly located, boomed. Bell Aircraft developed America's first jet in a building at the corner of Main and Rodney; the region itself became the capital of the country's aircraft industry. Bethlehem Steel roared just south of town in Lackawanna. Then came peace. The war contracts disappeared, just like that. Curtiss-Wright, which had made thousands of its famed P-40 fighters in Buffalo, said it didn't need the space and left for Columbus, Ohio, taking Dad's traffic job with it, if it even still existed. Trico appears not to have been an option, either. I can see Dad getting another "Genny," sitting in Nana's kitchen, trying to make it what it used to be. But Buffalo's once overflowing job market had drained into the lake. This is where he had come in.

He banged around for a couple of months before signing on with Remington Rand, in traffic management, by now a true career choice. Serendipity remains in this. On the day he was born, the *Buffalo Evening News* ran a small story on the front page with the headline: "Traffic Managers of Buffalo Organize." Dad was a native son in a city that owed its existence to traffic—the movement of goods, starting with grain—from the west on the Great Lakes, to the east through the Erie Canal (and later the railroad). Then in 1959, a completed Saint Lawrence Seaway bypassed Buffalo, and once and for all the city fell from the grand heights it had once occupied. Of course, by then Red McKee was long gone. Maybe he saw it coming. Or maybe if Helen O'Neil hadn't left for New York

City he would have stuck around. But Mom had left, and Dad had to get out. He was still sleeping in the attic. Aunt Alice remembers Dad once declaring after the war that 231 had become "a mausoleum." Nana hit the roof over that one.

She could be formidable, my grandmother. The impression I have is that Nana's parents were rather distant, quite displeased, as they saw it, that their daughter had rushed into marriage with a Pennsylvania coal-cracking itinerant plasterer, forcing him to settle down. Dad was a storyteller, but he had never said anything about his grandparents. Nana's relationship with her siblings appears to have been strained as well. And no surprise here, early on she was no fan of Mom's, either. Aunt Alice remembers the day Dad announced he was transferring to New York, and the chill that settled over the house.

Of course as a kid I knew none of this. Nana was just . . . my nana. Her annual weeklong visit to York was a hugely anticipated event by Kathy and me. In preparation Dad would take the legs off the foot of Kathy's bed, using the legs in the middle as a fulcrum to prop up the ones at the head with books. Nana had to sleep on an incline to aid her breathing. She was fun and witty, with a great cackle of a laugh. A sharp card player, she fit in well with the York moms' afternoon bridge club.

I don't think Nana ever expected to be a widow at age forty-seven, her husband dead of a heart attack. When that happened, she threw it all on Dad. I do think she and Dad grew closer, after a fashion, once Dad got some space between them. Mom says that as for the two of them, she and Nana affected first a truce and then a genuine affection, and she became a third daughter. This is saying something. Janie and A, *they* could have been twins; to her great credit, Nana saw to that. As for the man Nana married, it was said he had a nickname prior to their wedding: "Jack the Ripper," bestowed in honor of his wild nights. We have no way to verify this. But we do know this: Few people remember him even drinking at all after he married Anna Carey, a bookkeeper from Buffalo's Lower West Side.

———

Years ago, Kathy and I were talking about Cole Steel Equipment Company, about how its presence—its mere existence, really—dominated our lives because it so dominated Dad's. We put together a time line and were stunned to realize that Dad worked at Cole Steel in York for barely fifteen years, from 1954 to 1969. It was flabbergasting. That was all? Cole Steel and Dad, Dad and Cole Steel. The two had for us existed forever as one entity. Cole Steel had just always been, always in the present tense: Dad works at Cole Steel. This awful place he drives off to every morning.

Cole Steel manufactured metal office furniture. It was based in New York, where Dad first worked for them, but its York plant was a major player, and a major York employer, with operations at five sites in its best years. It made and shipped everything you could possibly imagine a working office would need. For a time in the late 1950s it also made portable typewriters, endorsed in advertisements by John Cameron Swayze, the famed newscaster. But mainly it was desks, chairs, filing cabinets and all the rest, in a mind-boggling array of combinations. In a

115-page Cole catalog from 1965, for instance, the "Futuric V Line" main desk comes in five sizes, with five different drawer possibilities. The add-on "L" section is available in nine different lengths and eleven separate drawer options. This was Dad's job: to keep track of every piece that came into or went out of his warehouse, with hundreds, even thousands, of the same item at any given time. Because of this, Cole Steel demanded that we McKees observe not four seasons in a year, but six. Autumn, winter, spring, and summer, plus "inventory" and "camping."

Inventory was the final week of July, six days of humid hell when Dad was required to have every item in the warehouse counted, by hand. The math was unmerciful: total desks and office chairs and filing cabinets shipped from the warehouse added to what still remained inside needed to equal exactly the total pieces that had been manufactured across Loucks Mill Road and moved into the warehouse via the buckets of the overhead conveyors. Dad would station two men in each designated area, then with his number two man they worked their way from location to location, totaling it all up. Once he kept coming up thirty units short in a place where card files were kept. So Dad and his number two started pulling the units out by themselves, only to discover that inside where the thirty cartons should have been there was instead an open space that some workers had turned into a sneak-off sleep area.

The carrot at the end of the inventory stick was the first two weeks of August—vacation!—when we always went camping. For years we celebrated Kathy's August 9 birthday at one or another of a state or national campground under the big brown tarp that Dad had strung—sometimes engineered—by employing some combination of available trees, spare tent poles, and as many feet of rope as was necessary to complete the architecture.

Dad loved everything about camping. Everything. From packing our supplies on his homemade roof rack (the weight balanced and secured under the tarp by the miles of rope he would need at the campsite) to setting up the tent to seasoning the big iron skillets over an open fire to getting that tarp erected over the picnic table exactly so.

He was in thrall to the stuff of camping. Coleman equipment, always Coleman. He had a hand-pumped "white gas" lantern with a socklike mantle, and to get it lighted he had to sort of blow the thing up. *KA-FWOOM! Still got the hair on my knuckles!* I was terrified the year he replaced the single-mantle with a double. But most especially he was enamored of his collapsible canvas water bucket. First of all, it collapsed, which rendered it merely ideal for packing purposes. When filled it expanded and the water would soak through, wherein lay its genius. The slow evaporation of the water, Dad announced each year (as if we'd never heard this before), kept the rest of the water cool. I never did figure out the science. And with that he'd set out to find the perfect tree branch from which to suspend his bucket, off by itself so that it "captured the air." Once, with the bucket securely elevated, the water seeping through, we climbed into the car for an excursion. But as we were pulling out, Dad suddenly stopped the car. "Look at that bucket," he exclaimed, pointing. "Cool water when we get back!"

Our first trip was to Tennessee and the Smoky Mountains when I was still in diapers (old-fashioned cloth—no small point of pride for Mom, surviving that). Our last was to Trap Pond State Park in Delaware in 1968. We once headed north to Algonquin National Park in Ontario. For Dad the fisherman, Canada was the Holy Grail. There were two trips to Acadia National Park in Maine, one taken with the Flick family—four adults and eight kids total in two cars towing pop-up trailers. We drove fourteen hours the first day, then headed up to Newfoundland the second week.

Often our vacations culminated with a night or two at Little Pine State Park in north-central Pennsylvania. We'd been everywhere, we liked to say, and yet the best place was only ninety miles away, northwest of Williamsport, just another state park. We found it by accident—maybe that's why we liked it so much, *we owned it*. Dad, a Pied Piper, at one time or the other got the McEntees, Schmitts, Mastersons, and Philbins as well as the Flicks to join him up there in the Appalachian Mountains under the pines in the Tiadaghton State Forest.

Little Pine is a magnificent place. Eastern white pines, straight as telephone poles and just as bare, disappear into the sky. In the age of sail these trees were prized as ship masts; now, their branches form a thick canopy seventy, eighty feet overhead. Sunshine, barely penetrating, dapples a soft carpet of brown pine needles. The surrounding land was originally settled by the English family, and in a small corner of the park rests the English family graveyard; a few of the worn, chipped tombstones date to the mid-1800s. The ground by the graves was always soft and loamy; you could push your fist in past your elbow, if you dared, sometimes hitting something hard, or so we thought. Everywhere the light was muted, the noises muffled. The only sound was of wind gently rushing far above. I have returned three times with Patrick. It is as spiritual a place as I have ever known.

On our old campfire nights—ritualized, stylized events with popcorn and s'mores and the singing of the old standards from Mom's generation—before the fire went out Dad would at some point in the week tell his story of "The White Deer." In it a young father goes hunting in winter to feed his starving family. He encounters a white deer. Nervous in the presence of such a spectacular specimen, his aim betrays him and his arrow barely wounds it in the left hind leg. For days (or weeks! or months! depending upon the telling Dad gave it) the hunter follows a track of blood in the snow, over mountains, across raging torrents, through deep valleys. Finally, he comes upon a cottage in a clearing, with red drops leading up the steps. The hunter knocks hesitantly on the door. A beautiful woman with skin as white as a cloud appears. He explains his journeys. The ravishingly gorgeous woman offers him dinner, and with that she turns, and with *that* the hem of her long skirt swirls and lifts a wee bit, revealing on her left ankle a white bandage . . . soaked with a bit of blood.

There Dad always ended, cryptically, ominously. Sometimes he told it in barely a minute, other times he took much longer, embellishing and extending. Looking back, the length he allotted was probably in direct proportion to how quickly he wanted to get into his sleeping bag. Long or short, between the graham crackers, marshmallows, and chocolate, and a forehead baked by the fire, for us "The White Deer" was always magical, the mysterious ending perfect.[1]

Finally, camping means Tommy Downey. He was maybe the best friend I ever had. For sure he was the big brother I never had. Mr. Downey worked for Republic Car Loading. He was in traffic management, too. He and Dad probably met at the York Traffic Club, a fraternity where the like-minded could commiserate about how the sales guys made promises that couldn't be kept and how the bosses never understood that conveyor belts break down. Dad ignored his strictest rule—never socialize with business associates—and he and Mr. Downey became fast friends. "Father," they called each other Father. An added bonus, Mom and Mrs. Downey hit it off terrifically. Their daughter, Anne, was three years older than Kathy; Tommy was four years older than I. In the late 1950s, early 1960s, our families ate Christmas dinner together, and even after the Downeys moved to New Jersey, Tommy continued to go camping with us, to Ontario and Maine, and, of course, Little Pine.

Tommy Downey occupies a singular, treasured place in my life. We have seen each other occasionally over the years, but

---

1. *The White Deer* is a 1945 novella by James Thurber. Dad, a voracious reader, may have cadged from it. I read it for the first time recently, with great trepidation. There is a white deer that becomes a princess; there are three hunters; there is a magical forest. But there is no white deer that becomes a beautiful woman with a bandage on her ankle; the hunters are fanciful and Thurberesque, not serious and single-minded; and there is no life-or-death quest for food. Best of all, there is no wondrously mysterious ending.

it was a full fourteen years before we caught up to each other for the first time after Dad died. College, marriage; me in Alaska, him in Colorado. Any number of obstacles had conspired against us. Then, in November 1983, I was in Denver and gave him a call. I ended up snowed in at his house for two days. But in all that time we barely spoke of Dad, our conversations instead sticking close to a filling-in of everything that had happened since. Not until Tom was driving me to the bus station, the roads finally cleared, did we shine a light on this darkened space. Tom told me how much those camping trips meant to him then. More important, how much more they meant now. Red McKee—Tommy and Anne always called Mom and Dad by their first names—had been his Confirmation sponsor. He said he became a fly fisherman because of Dad. He said Dad was one of the most influential people ever in his life. Then he stopped talking, and we rode the rest of the way in silence.

Had Dad still been alive that trip to the bus station would have been different, casual and regular. We could have continued talking—about our camping years, laughing about fishing with Dad, the two of us stripping naked to jump off the rocks, Dad angling as far from us as he could get. We could have remembered deer "hunting," when Dad would load me and Tommy and Kathy into the car after dinner and we'd drive the back roads with flashlights to our foreheads, trying to get our eyes "inside the beam," as Dad said, hoping double-red spots of deer retina would freeze in the light. But with Dad not here such conversations were impossible. It struck me like a thunderbolt: Tommy Downey exists for me—then and forever—in a world in which my father isn't dead. Because I have no substantive memory of him that doesn't include Dad still alive. There is for me no other person in my life like Tommy Downey.

Camping. I could talk of it forever. They were the best two weeks. Unfortunately, the other fifty belonged to Cole Steel. And whatever benefit Dad banked during his fourteen days away, he paid it back immediately on that first Monday back.

Stress does strange things to a body. Stress can raise blood pressure, which can tax the heart, make it overwork. Stress might make high cholesterol even worse, though what might really be the cause is the extra doughnuts eaten by way of finding relief from it. Or, as in Dad's case, the next (and the next and the next . . .) cigarette. Stress in many ways isn't a bad thing. It is the reason we as a species still exist. Stress hormones kick in to alert us when the surrounding environment is out to get us. We use those hormones to survive, or else. Cole Steel was Dad's environment.

Dad hated his job. No, that's unfair. Dad loved what he did for a living. He just hated where he did it. Actually that's unfair as well, if closer to the truth. Dad was the boss of the warehouse. He parked his car in the morning in his reserved space next to a nondescript entry door, walked up two flights of stairs to his office, a jumbled, overworked space as unimpressive looking as the front door. But through a wall of windows he could see into his warehouse—the conveyor belts, the boxes stacked to the ceiling, the men in the forklifts, the long row of loading docks in the front, the railroad track coming in the back. It was a state-of-the-art facility, a 3-D puzzle before there were such things, with lots of moving parts. Orders in, orders out. He loved it.

But what makes or breaks a job isn't what you do or where you do it. It's whom you do it for. That's what Cole Steel taught me. One of Dad's superiors was Otto Lewin, a vice president and general manager when Dad arrived in 1954. Dad worshiped the ground Mr. Lewin walked on, almost literally. On Sunday mornings when we drove to St. Joseph Church, one route took us past Mr. Lewin's house on Elmwood Boulevard. Dad would all but genuflect as he rode past.

Mr. Lewin had received a doctorate in economics from the University of Vienna. He was a half-owner of a company that made wood stoves when, in March 1938, Hitler annexed Austria in the infamous *Anschluss*. Nazis and rioters took to the streets, attacking Jews. Mr. Lewin's sister and her entire family were murdered. The next day Mr. Lewin was arrested and taken first to Buchenwald and then to Dachau concentration camp. Another sister in France somehow procured visas for him and a brother, but when Mr. Lewin returned to Vienna he decided to go to England, arranging to travel to the English Channel in a sealed railroad car. He made it to England only days before Germany invaded Poland on September 1, 1939.

His organizational skills in a refugee camp brought him to the attention of the British military and eventually to New York City, where he married and found work at a company called Bridge Metal. In short order, Bridge was bought by Masell Company, and Mr. Lewin was promoted to manager. Masell Manufacturing, as it would be known, eventually became a wholly owned subsidiary of Cole Steel Equipment. It was he, for the most part, who convinced Cole to move its furniture-making operations out of the city, and he was instrumental in getting Masell to purchase the rundown site of York Safe & Lock on Loucks Mill Road, where he moved operations in 1949. This makes Otto Lewin the reason we McKees lived in York.

He should have been a rather unprepossessing man, short and rotund as I recall, except he wasn't. He had a full head of wiry white hair that announced his arrival. He always drove a Chrysler, one of those grand mid-1950s elongations that must have taken twenty minutes to park. Kathy and I would see him now and again around York and declare: "There goes Mr. Lewin!"

From what I can gather (and remember from Dad), Mr. Lewin ran his company benevolently if a bit paternalistically, not unmindful of his own experiences. His nickname at Cole was "Pappy," though I doubt if to his face. He would sometimes show up to watch the Cole-sponsored softball team, the game being an immensely popular industrial-league pastime in south-central Pennsylvania. And he hired Negroes (and Jews and Poles and Germans and Italians—pronounced EYE-talians then) ahead of most. There is a story told that he once diffused a contentious management-labor confrontation by walking into a crowd of workers to promise a chicken dinner for everyone's family if they "went back in." They did, and he delivered on the dinner.

It was a couple of the men farther down the ladder but higher up on the food chain than Dad who chewed on him.

One was expert at keeping his underlings jumping in the air simply because he had the authority to make them jump. Dad was still the dutiful son, the loyal brother—his allegiance now to Mr. Lewin—and these guys knew how to use it against him. One of Dad's fishing buddies told me of a time when Dad called him once from out of the blue, during the day. Most unusual; the York dads at work existed apart in worlds of their own. This dad worked at a tire-retread company. My Dad was up against it, he said. One of his forklifts had lost some of its tire, the solid-rubber tread, and Dad could afford neither the time nor the situation of a downed forklift. "He was afraid to tell his boss about this tire," he says. "I sent my foreman down, and he patched it up. I'm only surmising here, but he just had to get it fixed and keep the boss from knowing." It's no way to have to run a business.

Dad was a bit of a martyr, too, and Cole was the wrong place to be one of those. Maybe any workplace is. He had convinced himself, I think, that it couldn't run without him. He had to be there. One year a bunch of the York Crowd families organized a weekend excursion to the cabins at Worlds End State Park, another piece of God's country in north-central Pennsylvania. Dad picked up Kathy and me from school at 3:00 P.M., a full three hours and fifteen minutes ahead of his normally rigid schedule. For that one day the sun stood still.

Cole Steel dictated the theater of our nightly dinner. "How was your day, dear?" was no ironically asked cliché at the McKee table. Dad came home with his whistle at 6:15 P.M. He had two beers. When we lived on Wilshire Drive he would stand in the kitchen by the back door and read the *York Dis-*

patch, the evening paper. Once dinner started, Kathy and I knew not to talk. There wasn't tyranny in this; we just knew the first portion of dinner belonged to Dad. He used it to tell Mom—in great detail—exactly how his day had been.

The shipping orders from New York were waiting for him when he got in at 8:30. Dad had first to ascertain if what he needed was actually in the warehouse. The production guys had told New York it was, but production always told New York that. Dad, with his number two, would route the goods by carrier—Dad favored Motor Freight Express—and then figure which diverse orders could be combined in the same trucks. "Drop shipments," these were called. The wheels needed to be set in motion quickly because New York rang him up midmorning. *Are the orders out?* That put Dad on the phone for hours—explaining, finessing, cajoling (and flat-out lying, I'm sure). He couldn't ship what he didn't have, but New York didn't hear him. *Production says you got it.* So it went the rest of the day. Stuff sitting in the warehouse was money not being made. *Get it out.* Truckers were late spotting their rigs on the dock. The railroad didn't send enough cars.

Dad's bosses also made regular, dark appearances in these recountings. They'd show up in the warehouse unannounced and change everything. And then on occasion Dad would relate a particularly dramatic episode, like, say, when a two-drawer file cabinet or some such piece had fallen off the conveyor belt and smashed to the floor, barely missing one of Dad's guys, spewing ball bearings all over the floor, bringing it all to a halt. This conversation with Mom lasted perhaps twenty minutes. And it was a conversation. Mom knew the players, the ongoing story. This was *her* job. She knew when to jump in with a well-timed *"hmm," "uh-huh,"* or correctly asked question to push the narrative along. Eventually Dad talked himself off the ledge for another day, and he would turn his attention to us.

Mom tells her own story about Dad's boss, about one of the men who made him miserable. She was with Dad at this boss's house for one of those awful work-related pretend social affairs that everybody hates. On this occasion it was just the four of them, Mom and Dad and Mr. and Mrs. Boss. At the appropriate moment when the men were to talk, the wife took Mom on what Mom supposed would be a tour of the showcase house. "But all she showed me was her linen closet," Mom says. The various towels and wash cloths and sheets and pillow cases, they were all meticulously rolled and folded and arranged by size, color, and texture, cross-filed to within an inch of their lives. The exactness was breathtaking. For Mom it was the moment early in the horror movie when the unsuspecting guest suddenly realizes she is trapped by a host who is utterly, certifiably insane.

About once a month Dad went to the warehouse on Saturday morning. I often went with him, under strict orders to be seen and not heard, to speak only when spoken to, to present a firm handshake and look the man right in the eye. On these days Dad did not wear his shirt and tie. Paint-spattered khaki pants and flannel shirt sufficed. Once there, however, he never seemed to do much. He'd throw his coat on the chair of his office and head straight away to the floor and just walk around, stopping to talk with whoever was in picking up overtime. Dad bought them coffee from the brew-a-cup machines in the center of the warehouse. He always bought the coffee. It was lousy, lukewarm dishwater—they all said so—but apparently that didn't matter. Dad had loaded his pockets with change before leaving the house. Whether the cup plopped down right side up or not, it gave him something to talk about across the boss-worker divide.

Dad ended his Saturday over at the loading docks to talk with the truckers. Dad envied the truckers. He had been one. In a different world he might still have been one. Like a baseball manager who knows he is only as good as his players, Dad knew he was only as good as the men driving the trucks. When we were on the road at night Dad always flashed his high beams a couple of times when a trucker passed him and wanted to move in. Dad was one with every trucker on the road. They were keeping America moving. Maybe this driver here who had just flashed his lights back at Dad by way of thanks was carrying a Cole Steel load. Dad needed his warehouse workers, the foremen, the forklift guys, and the loaders. But at the other end of the line it was the truckers who showed up on time with the trailer of four-drawer letter files, a Cole Steel staple, to make Red McKee look good. "Modern-day cowboys," Dad called them, out there on the open road, their own boss. I think he envied that freedom, real or imagined.

I always sensed in Dad a certain yearning. A wistfulness that maybe his life could have turned out . . . not better, just differently. Some of this, perhaps most of this, was the product of the job situation, the boss situation. But not all of it. Dad never had the luxury of career options. Had he, he might have become a forest ranger. He talked of that sometimes, and he enjoyed chatting them up when we were in the national parks. He also talked about going back to Australia, where he had been during the war. About going back maybe even to live, him and Mom, to retire there after Kathy and I were out of college. It's what America's Wild West must have been like during the late nineteenth century, he said, adhering closely to his truck-driving cowboy theme.

Interviewing Mom and Dad's friends for this book, I learned something. "Your Dad talked to me several times about starting our own company," Mr. Masterson said. "He had a definite idea in mind. He had it worked out to where there was a particular position for me. He quoted me a salary. He had a business plan of what he was going to need and who he was going to need. He had to have given this some serious thought. It had to do with traffic—logistics, warehousing, distribution. Maybe all of it thrown into one."

Mr. Masterson said Dad talked to him three or four times. Nothing heavy, always light, but it also wasn't mere we-oughta-start-a-business chatter over a few beers. Mr. Masterson always said no. He had six kids by then and a very good situation where he was. Dad came back a couple of times. "He had dreams of something," Mr. Masterson said. "Something he wanted to do on his own, or on our own. There was clearly something in the back of his mind. Something he wanted to create."

I don't think Dad was dissatisfied with his life, nor that he was unhappy. I think he was happy, at least mostly. What happened, I believe, is that he learned what we all learn, eventually, that no life turns out like we want it to. It just doesn't. But you also learn—if you're lucky—that that's all right. Because there's no way it could have anyway.

I understood this yearning. Even more, I absorbed it and acted on it. When I graduated from Allentown College of St. Francis de Sales in Pennsylvania in 1974, I wanted to get as far away from everything as I could. To go see it for myself, whatever "it" was, wherever "it" was. My first choice was Australia. I don't recall this as a conscious attempt to complete Dad's unfinished business. Down Under was just very far away. But I had no idea how to get there. So instead I applied to Vista—Volunteers in Service to America, the domestic Peace Corps—with the hope of being sent somewhere, anywhere. Vista turned me down. I realize now (only now) that I was likely the last thing they needed: another gung-ho liberal arts major with no hands-on skill and zero practical experience. I should have paid attention to Dad out there at the farm. I had no Plan B.

There can be no bigger loser on a college campus than the graduate who returns to take more classes, hang in the cafeteria, see if he can still score with the new crop of freshman girls. That was me the ensuing spring semester at Allentown College. Ostensibly there to get my teacher's certification, in truth I had nowhere else to be. I had by then set my sights on Alaska through the Jesuit Volunteer Corps or a teaching position at a high school in the Virgin Islands. But with no word from either and summer under way, I took a teaching job at a Catholic high school in the Harrisburg diocese. There had been a time in my life when that would have been the dream job, but not now. I signed on reluctantly. When both the Jesuit Volunteer Corps and the Virgin Islands then came through in the same week late in July, I was devastated.

I had no choice. I had to get out of the teaching job and get to Alaska, my preferred destination. Actually, I did have choices, and perhaps that's the point. Dad's years of sweating Cole Steel had provided me a middle-class life, and with it options he never had. Though he died when I was a senior in high school, the foundation was solidly in place for me to go to college. Once I graduated, however adrift, there were few doors that weren't still open, if only I could push through them. Dad made sure I could do what he never could: pretty much whatever I wanted. And what I wanted, maybe needed, was Alaska.

The high school I had signed on with had taken a tumble in recent years, and the priest in charge had been brought in that very summer to bring it back. He had big plans, and I was to be one of his boys, part of his new guard on the ground floor, an English teacher and junior-varsity basketball coach. Indeed, I had been handpicked. This priest knew me. He had been a parish priest at St. Joe's. I'd served Mass for him; he had watched me grow up. When I'd go to Confession to him, kneeling in the dark and talking to the black screen, I knew he recognized my voice. He had to know I knew, too, even as we both pretended otherwise. My request to void my contract was a personal affront, an embarrassing black mark on his record before his first school year had even started. When I went back to plead my case, the secretaries in the office avoided looking at me, kept their eyes on the papers on their desks.

He could have made me stay. Legally, he had the right. But he didn't. He understood. He also knew I couldn't do the year and then rethink it. That would have been a reasonable request, not to mention the honorable course on my part. But a lot can happen in a year, and he knew that too. I sat across from him in his office, at another large wooden desk. As a young man, he told me, he had arranged to be stationed in Africa. But his mother had asked him not to go, not yet, to wait awhile. She was getting older and wanted him close to home. He postponed going and then, of course, never got there. He had put together a successful career as a priest in the Diocese of Harrisburg. He was held in such esteem by the bishop as to be his man to turn this thing around. But sometimes he wondered what might have been, what had never been. He stood up. He put his hands on my shoulders. "Go," he said. "Go."

Getting to Alaska changed everything for me. I have Dad to thank for that. Mom helped, too. She thinned her lips, squared her jaw, and let me go without making my leaving about her being left alone. She had seen too much of that, perhaps, with Dad and Nana. And she had once wanted out herself. I spent two years—1975 to 1977—in the Jesuit Volunteer Corps, teaching at St. Mary's Mission, an Eskimo-Indian boarding school in southwest Alaska on the Andreafsky River just north of the Yukon River, about ninety miles from the Bering Sea. In 1978, Noreen D'Ottavio and I married on July 8 in York and then drove back to Alaska in a five-year-old Fiat. Noreen and I had met not long before I left for Alaska. On our first date she beat me at miniature golf. Most of that summer was shadowed by the fact that I was leaving. She always told me that I should go, that I had to go. My first year at St. Mary's, like Dad during World War II, I lived for the letters. The second year, Noreen joined the JVC and came to the mission. After we married, we moved to Fairbanks and lived there until 1982.

People ask sometimes, "Why Alaska?" The long answer is all of the above. My short, flip answer is also true. Alaska is where I went to be young and stupid. Everyone needs a place to be young and stupid, and in Alaska I succeeded fabulously on both counts. I was, first, a volunteer, paid twenty-five dollars a month, eschewing the business-career ethos. I also planned to save the world by the end of the week. My God, was I full of myself! I learned big lessons at St. Mary's, ones I carry with me still. I couldn't save the world, for one thing. For another, what makes something, anything, so good (at St. Mary's I was in the middle of nowhere and surrounded always by the same people) is also what makes it so difficult. One comes with the other; deal with it. I have come to apply that lesson to all facets of my life. And I know what it feels like to walk into a room and be the only person in it who looks like me. Everyone should experience that.

Mostly, though, Alaska freed me of regret. This is a terrific feeling, and I owe it to Dad directly. He made sure that I made sure to have no regrets.

Two no-regret Alaska stories.

(One) The state was just beginning to build local high schools out in the villages. Basketball programs were starting, too, and word got out that I'd played some. Soon enough the local school districts were paying for another volunteer and me to fly around with a bush pilot to referee weekend tournaments. That was cool enough. But one set of games was in Mountain Village northwest of St. Mary's on the Yukon River. Some of the men from Mountain came up and loaded us into a sled on the back of their snow machine. I was in the sled, the other ref was on the runners, and we took off. Suddenly he started pounding me on the shoulder and screaming, "Everyone we went to college with is sitting behind a desk right now, but we are on the fucking Yukon Trail at thirty-five below zero!"

(Two) The summer of 1977, Noreen and I stayed at the mission and worked construction. I drove a dump truck for the state; Noreen worked as a cook for a crew putting in new electrical at St. Mary's airport. In September a Jesuit priest and a pilot offered to fly us both to Fairbanks if we first spent two weeks with him flying to his parishes in Alaska's Athabascan Indian interior to help winterize various parish buildings. We flew to Kaltag at night, guided to the gravel airstrip by rows of garbage cans filled with fire. On the ground we met our air-traffic controller, one Edgar Kallands. In 1925 he had been the second musher in the famed sled-dog relay that brought the diphtheria serum to a desperate Nome. To live in Alaska is to know these stories. Noreen and I earned our keep those ten days—renailing corrugated tin roofs, pumping heating oil, painting, whatever. On one trip, a few thousand feet above a brown Yukon, the birch trees a golden yellow, the tundra a burnt-red brick, our priest-pilot declared deviously: "Let's take a look at the water." With that he stood his twin-engine plane on its nose and took it straight down, not bringing the wings up until we were maybe ten feet over the water. The banks of the Yukon were above us now, and that's how we took it home, snaking the river.

========

They say that if you cut down a tree and take off in the same direction that it's falling, that no matter what size the tree or how fast you run you won't get out from underneath it, that it will always crash on top of you. True or not, that's me and Cole Steel.

I sprinted from the very idea of a career in business, the one thing of all things that Dad was so grateful to run to. So grateful in fact that he was willing to work himself to death on its behalf. And I cannot be convinced to the contrary. In college I disdained the economics majors. I was an English major. I walked around with a paperback book stuck in my back pocket, making sure the top inch was well visible. I played on the basketball team; I appeared in some student-directed plays produced by the theater department. Yes, I fancied myself quite the latter-day Renaissance man. I was going to "teach"; I was going to "write." I aspired not to a career, but a calling.

For me the math has forever been unforgiving: Career equals death. All those years watching Dad at the blackboard of the dinner table and the quotient calculates the same no matter how I figure it. I think sometimes of Jim Calhoun, the men's basketball coach at the University of Connecticut. At age fifteen, while playing center field, a guy on the other side of the fence yelled to him that he needed to go home because his father had just died of a heart attack. When Jim Calhoun's father had been fifteen years old, he had heard much the same callous shout while walking down a street in East Boston. And yet Coach Calhoun chose the pressure cooker of a big-time college basketball career. How? Why? No way I was going to kill myself packing boxes into a truck. Spend my life on the phone talking to New York. Allow a boss to dominate the conversation at my dinner table. I would not be my father.

At my job at the *Wall Street Journal* I don't hire and I don't fire. I don't do inventory. There are many of me, perhaps thirty such copy editors on the Global Copy Desk. The story comes to me. I edit, write the headline, and move it along. I work to a deadline every night and when it's over, it's over. There is nothing to cart home, nothing to worry about, nothing even to talk about. Indeed, after the rush it can be difficult even to remember what I did. When I take a vacation, none of it comes with me. I am completely replaceable. And while I am responsible to a boss, no one is responsible to me. None of this is by accident. There also isn't any stress, despite (or because of) the tyranny of deadline. Prior to the *Journal* my experience had been in magazines. To take what in that world consumes months and compress it into a single workday seemed unfathomable to me. But immediately I recognized that the tyranny of deadline *removes* the pressure. The first edition must be out the door at 7:30. Therefore, it will be. I am sure there are stressful jobs at the *Journal*. I just don't think mine is one of them. That may be the trick itself.

My one foray into management was . . . not successful. I knew it was a mistake to accept the offer even as I was saying yes to it. No surprise, I didn't work out. I was the first sports editor of the new *Weekend Journal*, an every-Friday addition to the paper. Gone was the daily deadline. Suddenly the work didn't have to be done that night. There was no closing bell. The aggravation, whatever benefit to my "career," was not worth it. All I had ever wanted was a good job. I'd had one and left it. When an opportunity to return to the copy desk materialized, I gladly demoted myself.

Career equals death. Business equals death. I am aware of the irony of my working at the *Wall Street Journal*. That I got there at all was pure dumb luck. In that regard so has been my entire professional life. It begins of course with my middle-class existence, courtesy of Dad. I never had a financial worry, ever. I always knew I would go to college. Going to college meant I wasn't exposed to the draft and Vietnam. My freshman class was the last year afforded the student deferment. In my draft-lottery year, 1971, November 17 came up No. 298. I wasn't going, and as it turned out no one in my draft year of 1973 went anyway. That was the year the draft was abolished. In 1978, I married Noreen D'Ottavio. That makes me lucky on all counts, including that Noreen is a recently retired owner of an investment company. So I'm not trying to kid anyone here, take any credit not due me: I never had a career because I never needed one. I know how lucky I have been.

Even when I should have had to worry I didn't have to worry. That summer after our JVC experience, when Noreen and I worked construction, we made so much money it was silly. That was 1977, the first heady days of the Alaska pipeline, and wages had gone crazy. Tack on twenty hours–plus of time and a half a week, and we made enough not to have to work for the next twelve months. We traveled the United States, back-packed Europe for sixty days on a rail pass. I then returned to Paris on my own to try out for a lower-division basketball team. Failed at that, I called Noreen on a transatlantic phone and asked her to marry me. In that predigital age such calls still held romance. I didn't just dial her up. I had to go to an international call center and sign some forms before being shown to a private booth. *Noreen?* Steve. *We should get married.* It was all very Cary Grant. We married that July and drove back to Alaska, where we both got good-paying jobs. Of course.

As for the *Journal*, I should never have been hired. Surely not by any objective employment standard or résumé. It's not just that I had never worked for a daily newspaper before. Avoiding a career takes its own brand of hard work. In the ten years before landing feet first at the *Journal*, I'd knocked around writing two books, put in a couple of years as a copy editor at a health magazine, spent nearly three years as a stay-at-home dad, and in the eleven months immediately prior had been a jack of all trades editor/writer for a slate of micro-niche men's fitness magazines.

I applied to the *Journal* twice, the first time in 1986— without ever having made a professional copyediting mark in my life. I did well enough on the test for the supervisor to take my results to the next level where, he assured me, he would be laughed out of the room for suggesting such a raw hire. I applied again in 1994, armed with my on-again, off-again

copyedit work at the women's magazine and a first few months
at the men's magazine. This new supervisor didn't mind that I
had been through this before and gotten nowhere. I passed
the test again. He said keep in touch. Five months passed before he called. Maybe I got something, he said.

Now the lucky part, or maybe the luckiest part. I don't run
into this particular supervisor at this exact moment (he would
move to a new position in a few months), and I don't get hired
at the *Wall Street Journal*. I believe that as firmly as I do that
Dad's job killed him.

We were the same age, early forties. He had grown up outside Philadelphia, and we bonded over stories of the Philadelphia Catholic League. Most of the guys I'd played basketball
with at Allentown College were from the Philly Catholic
League. He had no business hiring me. I knew that. Surely he
knew that. And yet he did. Then he left his office. He said he'd
be awhile, to explain to his superior why bringing in a guy with
no newspaper experience was the smart move. In the meantime, he told me to fill out the official application, last job first
and all the rest. He returned chuckling—it had taken awhile,
as promised. "You're in," he said. I joked nervously that I always had a problem filling out applications. Too many gaps and
hard-to-explain lulls.

He turned suddenly serious. Listen here, chief, he said. He
was hiring me precisely because I couldn't fill it out. Because I
did go off to Alaska, volunteered to teach Eskimos in the middle of nowhere. Because I had written a couple of books, including one where I'd dropped everything and taken off for a

year to attend sports events. Because I'd spent an extended period with my son as a house dad.

"I want as diverse a copy desk as I can get," he said. He said he wanted young and old, black and white, men and women. Ambitious young lions who didn't know nothing except that they wanted to own the paper by the end of the week. Contented, wizened hands who had written headlines for the *Noah's Ark Dispatch*. Somewhere in all that, between all that, is where a copy desk finds its strength, he said. Where, he wasn't sure, but he believed firmly in its existence. He was hiring me to add to that muscle. He even liked that I hadn't gone to journalism school. Precisely what I'd bring to the table he didn't know, but he was willing to find out. "Someday," he said, "someone is going to have a question in a story and we're going to be on deadline and you'll be the one who knows the answer." He pointed to my résumé and its gaping white spaces. "One more thing," he said. "You work at the *Wall Street Journal* now. You'll never have this problem again." One last time, Dad took care of me.

———

I remain of conflicting minds about Dad and Cole Steel, Cole Steel and Dad. On the one hand, I think in some ways Cole was a good place to work, at least as workplaces go. There was Otto Lewin, for one. His demeanor permeated the place, even if not to every nook and cranny. Cole finally shuttered for good in 1990 when an employee stock-ownership plan was rebuffed by the owner at the time. It was called Cole Office Environments by then. Seven years later, nearly 300 former employees from both the labor and management aisles held a reunion. Read the newspaper accounts of the get-together and you constantly trip over the word "family" describing workers' deep-seated attachment to the place.

We experienced some of that. When Dad had his first heart attack in 1963, he was refinishing the basement. When he came upstairs, he left behind a half-done ceiling and countless details. Weeks later, once Dad was "out of danger," as the doctors gravely put it, we were able to ask whether the basement was in danger of remaining forever halved. On a following Saturday we received our answer. Six, eight, maybe ten men from Cole Steel—a few of Dad's executive peers, some of his warehouse floor men—came to the house with tool belts, power saws, and paint brushes and in a couple of cacophonous hours finished the place to the last tile.

So I have to believe that in at least a few ways Dad had a good thing going at Cole Steel. And if I believe that, I have to lay some of this back on him. His boss was a prick? Sure was, but who hasn't had a pain-in-the-ass boss? Get over it and move on. Stop with the martyr thing.

On the other hand, I know as a kid (and for many years after) I never gave Dad the credit he deserved for the job he did, the work he did. Back then it was about me. Of course it was about me. I was the kid and all Cole Steel did was make him miserable. I never allowed that he might have liked his job, or at least the work. That there had to be a creative component to it, a challenge to it. It wasn't just boxes in, boxes out.

There was art involved. Those drop-shipment trucks had to be packed backward, the last unit on being the first one off, the stuff coming from all corners of the warehouse, maybe ten, fifteen trucks in play simultaneously. He struck a deal on the cheap to fill up refrigerated railcars from California or Florida with Cole Steel stock so they wouldn't deadhead home. "Reefers," these were called. That saved the company millions, I've been told. All this could be satisfying, perhaps sometimes very. I never got that. Worse, what I completely missed then—and I shouldn't have, because I'd seen him in action on those Saturday mornings in the warehouse—is that to do his job well he had to treat his people well.

Once on a Friday night we were at the Phillie Cafe on West Philadelphia Street. We went there now and again for Maryland hard-shell crabs—up from Baltimore, crusted with rock salt and Old Bay seasoning. The Catholic Church's no-meat Friday and its call to sacrifice and denial was always lost on me, in part thanks to hard-shell crabs. They are eaten with your hands, your sleeves rolled up, salt and seasoning under your fingernails, shells and gunk mounding on the newspapers that cover the table and get soaked through. Keep the beer coming. Makes for a great night out.

There was Dad, right from work, so he was still in his white shirt and tie, attacking another crab. He loved his hard shells, enthusiastically learning the secrets of eating one. Break off the legs and the claws, then remove the key-shaped section on the underside. It's called the apron, but it looks like a key and, more to the point, it acts like one. Because once removed the top and bottom shells are easily unlocked, revealing the sweet meat in the body compartments. Crabs are hard work, more ritual than meal, but terrific fun and well worth it. Suddenly, the waitress appeared with a pitcher of beer for Mom and Dad, sodas for Kathy and me. "From the table over there," she said, pointing with her chin.

It was a group of men, no women. They worked in the warehouse, Dad said offhandedly. He gave them a brief nod, returned in like manner by the men. Do not stare, Dad commanded, and returned to his crabs. So of course I stared. They wore cut-off tees and work shirts. They were not wearing ties. That's what I noticed.

When the waitress put the bill on our table, Dad got her attention, pointed in the general direction of the men, and whispered to her. By now I was watching Dad closely and glancing furtively at the men whenever I could, aware that some intricately choreographed dance was unfolding. The waitress wrote some more on the bill and then handed it back to Dad. We got up. I thought Dad might go over and talk to the men, but no. He nodded again in their direction. They nodded back. With that, he paid the bill and we left.

Litton Industries bought Cole Steel in 1961. That did not bode well for Cole, or at least for Dad. Charles Litton, Sr., had founded the company in 1934, a pre-pre-Silicon Valley startup of sorts, to mass produce vacuum tubes. In 1953, Charles Bates "Tex" Thornton bought the company, kept the Litton name, and turned it into a multinational defense contractor. Thornton had been a Ford Motor Company "whiz kid"; he had worked for Howard Hughes. Under Thornton's tutelage, Litton became one of the great American postwar conglomerates—maybe the first one. He died in 1981, the year he was awarded the Medal of Freedom. But in 1961, when Litton bought Cole, Thornton relinquished the presidency, though he stayed on as chairman and became chief executive.

For a while, there was a burst of enthusiasm at Cole—"a division of Litton Industries," as trumpeted in the full-page ads that now appeared in the York city directories. But in 1963 the name of a Dad nemesis made its first appearance in the Cole listing. By 1968, Mr. Lewin's name was gone and in 1970 so were the ads, the Cole mention reduced to a pair of un-bolded lines. And by then Dad's trusted No. 2 had left the company to seek his own top spot. I have worked for the boss from hell, two of them. Career equals death. At my first opportunity I quit both, running and screaming from the room, my tail between my legs. How did Dad do it, work for bosses like that for all those years but not let it twist him into one as well?

After my freshman year in college in 1971, I worked as a playground director in an African-American section of the city of York. The first day we did all the getting-to-know-you games with the kids. On the second, a little boy with a big Afro came up to me and asked, "Are you John McKee's son?" The question came from nowhere and for a moment it struck me dumb. Finally I said I was. "My dad worked for your dad," the boy said and took off. On the third day a man came to the playground with the boy and walked directly to the pavilion where I was standing. "You're Steve McKee," he said. "John McKee's son." They were declaratory sentences, not interrogative, and in any event they were coming at me too quickly to respond. Well, he said, he was this little boy's father. He introduced himself. Then he said, "I just wanted to drop by to say hello and shake your hand."

From that I will take it that Dad was a good man.

WEDNESDAY,
OCTOBER 1; 7:00 P.M.

Mary Liz? Oh my god, it's Mary Liz.

I was standing in the flagstone foyer of the house. There because, well, I don't remember why. But while walking by the front door I looked out one of its three slit windows lined up in descending order, like a set of stairs. Maybe I glanced out because for a couple of hours now there had been people coming and going, bringing food and drink, a hug and some tears, and I couldn't get enough of it, of all of it.

So I looked out the window and there she was. *Mary Liz!* Of the people I might have expected to see out that window, Mary Liz was not one of them. What was she doing here? The answer—there could be only one answer—turned my world upside down. Meaning it was right side up again, at least for a moment. She was here to see me.

Mary Liz was not my girlfriend. Certainly not if you had asked her. I, on the other hand, had been wishing only that for months. I was desperately, foolishly, hopelessly in love with her. And there was no way she couldn't have known it. Now here she was, unbidden—that's what amazed me—walking up the driveway to my front door. She had on a blue blouse with white buttons, a light-brown suede jacket. We all had suede jackets. Blonde hair to her shoulders, pulled back off her face, a beautiful smile, blue eyes to fall into. She was tall, too, tall enough that the one time we had slow danced she was able to rest her head on my shoulder.

She was up the driveway, almost to the front porch. It was a slab of concrete with a crack running diagonally across it that drove Dad nuts when he had the whole thing replaced and it separated again on the same line. I opened the door and pushed on the screen, took one step outside, fighting the urge to run right to her. Mary Liz stopped when she saw me looking at her, and there we stood for a moment, on either side of Dad's line in the porch.

"Hi," I said, exhaling all of the past twenty-four hours in one short syllable.

What is it about high school and those four years that bend and shape in ways you can't forget and can never escape? For instance, will there ever be anyone more amazingly "cool" in your life than the seniors when you were a freshman? And not just when you were a freshman, but for the rest of your life. The way they seemed to invent everything right in front of your brand-new eyes—the pep rallies, the football cheers, that certain insouciance only they could affect when getting yelled at for goofing off in the hall between classes.

Everything about the York Catholic Class of 1967 left me agog my freshman year. They were a wild bunch, as I still re-member them, bringing an energy to the school that always seemed to teeter on the edge of chaos yet kept the entire place pumped and alive. Compounding it all was the fact that my sister, Kathy—"MUH-key," as she was called—was in that class. Kathy was in the color guard with the rest of the tall girls; their involvement and commitment had transformed the band front into major status, especially for a girl at York Catholic. Kathy smoked. She could go into a bar and get beer. She could drive fast, expertly double clutching the "three in the tree" on Dad's Chevy. She was a great dancer, maybe the best in the school. Though often she'd come to a dance for only a little while before heading out to someone's house to a real party, swearing me to secrecy. She was everything I was, and would remain, too terrified ever to be. If no one was cooler than the seniors, no senior was cooler than Kathy. Her position at York Catholic didn't gain me entry to the inner sanctum, but I was at least "McKee's Brother," an identity of sorts, if just barely.

Once, I had to deliver a message to Sister Anne Jerome's advanced-placement biology class at the far end of the school in Brady Science Hall. I knew Kathy was in there, along with the rest of the really smart kids, and that they'd be at the lab tables dissecting the cats. Sister Anne Jerome, surely the coolest nun in the school, ran a loose ship with her college-prep students, and when I walked in there were lots of jibes and snide remarks thrown my way, none of which I returned. (Are you kidding?) Red-faced, I delivered the note and scurried out. That night Kathy told Mom and Dad the story of how I had fumbled my way through the room. And how after I left, Joe Kochansky—"Jumpin' Joe Kochansky," senior basketball star!—shouted out to a howling class, "Hey, MUH-key, did you have any brothers who lived?" Then, as if to validate Kochan-sky's observation, I pointed out to a laughing Kathy and a Mom and Dad trying not to, that wait, yes, Kathy *did* have a brother who lived—you know, *me*. Mom and Dad burst after that.

My sophomore year Sister Regina Cecilia, the chorus and choir nun, staged a full-blown production of *Oklahoma!* A gutsy move from a great teacher. Until Sister Regina, an Im-maculate Heart of Mary nun, arrived at York Catholic my freshman year, the drama and music departments were not even points on the school's thermometer of cool. Quite the opposite, in fact, they were backwater, geeky pursuits gener-ally dismissed by the kids who somehow get ordained to make these decisions.

How does that happen, by the way? How is it some kids get chosen to set the high school agenda for everybody else? As we would have said back then, "Who died and left them boss?" But indeed they were the boss, the rest of us mere employees grateful for the work. My junior year a couple of the guys de-cided that everyone needed a theme song. So they went about assigning each of the juniors (or more likely, most of the jun-iors) his or her own "song." That way when we passed some-one in the hall between classes we could point to them and shout out the first couple of lines. Only two or three guys could have done that, handed out song titles—this one is *yours*, we say so—knowing that the rest of us would be thrilled to sing along. Mine was "Steve McKee's Got a Brand New Bag!" from the James Brown title of almost the same words. I have no idea why that song, or whether it mocked me or not. I was happy to be included.

You took your cool where you could, and held on to it. Once, even Dad got ordained as such. Until it happened, though, I would have thought it impossible. Other kids' parents could be cool, but your own? This was the same Dad who at my eighth-grade graduation dance from St. Joe's had, during the parents' dance, swept Mom up and waltzed grandly around the other parents, who at least had the decency to barely move and not mortify their kids. I could only be grateful he didn't get out there for the twist or the limbo, or, total humiliation, the Freddie—that silly thing from Freddie and the Dreamers wherein you kind of did jumping jacks in time to the music.

Dad got cool one Saturday night my sophomore year. I'd spent the day with Mike Kochansky (Joe's younger brother) and Tim Pfister at Rolling Acres, a pitch-and-putt golf course heading towards Muddy Creek. We walked the two and a half miles out, ran through fifty-four holes, and then hitchhiked back to my house for dinner, me and Mike and Tim and Mom and Dad. It was a great night, like I imagine it might once have been for Dad, sitting around the kitchen table at Nana's with the guys. Dad could be silly, loads of fun, and that night he pushed away Cole Steel and gave into it. At one point we were talking about Brian McDevitt. He had been one of the shortest kids in our class when we arrived at York Catholic, but just like that, it seemed, he had shot up. "Brian McDevitt grew a lot?" Dad yelled out. "Brian McDevitt grew a lot?" We all looked at him, no idea why this fact needed repeating. "Well," Dad declared, "that sure must make his Dad happy!" That brought everything to a dead halt. Dad was telling a joke. At least, it had sounded like he was telling a joke. But where was it, the joke? Dad started laughing his silliest, I-really-crack-myself-up cackle. "Brian McDevitt grew A LOT! I'll bet that makes his Dad happy . . . because his father's in real estate. Get it? *Brian McDevitt grew A LOT!*"

It was one of those embarrassing father-son moments in the presence of friends that should have had me crawling under the kitchen table. But the joke was so awful, and Dad had delivered it with such enthusiasm, that when we finally got it, such as it was, there was another sudden silence followed immediately by a hysterical why-are-we-laughing? howl. The next Monday at school Tim Pfister came up to me before first period. "Your dad is so cool," he said and then started laughing again. "Brian McDevitt grew a lot!" Tim was one of the guys who had handed out the song titles. And he had just declared my dad was cool.

York Catholic High School in the 1960s was an inviolate bastion of absolute maleness. Boys' sports and their testosterone ethos ruled. Football and basketball. Girl athletes didn't exist; cheerleaders did. When Sister Regina Cecilia came to the school and started a chorus, she didn't change that reality, but she did muscle her way into it. She started first by getting the captain of the football team on her side. A hard-nosed, boisterous, charismatic sort, he in turn recruited teammates. That brought on board other male unassailables, which—just like that—guaranteed the girls would sign up too. Sister Regina was tireless in her efforts—shaming some, cajoling others, and I think, tricking even more ("he said he'd join if you joined"). The next year she pulled out all the stops with *Oklahoma!*—

dancing and everything. An unheard-of undertaking, it succeeded only because Sister Regina defiantly ensured it be too good to be dismissed. With that she vaulted the spring musical into third place on the "Fightin' Irish" school calendar of must-do, must-see events. It provided no glorious season-long acclaim, as did football and basketball, but for one weekend, oh my.

I wasn't in *Oklahoma!* I was just another audience member at the freshman-sophomore show when Jeff Witman walked out for a curtain call after his star turn as Jud Fry, the doomed ranch hand. Jeff was a football player, a sophomore starter. He once decided that stupid, groaning puns were to be our class's form of humor, and the rest of us followed along. Like Tim and the others who assigned us song titles, only Jeff could have made stupid puns smart. So we showered Jeff in a thunderous standing ovation, the girls squealing. He stood there and let the applause rain upon him as if it were his birthright—which, in the grand scheme, it was. Standing with the rest of my classmates, I decided right there that next year I would be on that stage, washing myself in this acclaim. I was no star athlete, student council member, designated guy. I was a yearbook photographer. But maybe it could happen for me.

The spring musical my junior year was *Brigadoon*, the story of two American hunters who stumble upon a village in Scotland that appears once every one hundred years. Early in September I joined the chorus, sang in both the fall and Christmas presentations, had a blast. I also made sure to befriend Sister Regina. She had what I wanted, maybe needed: a starring role in *Brigadoon.* I got the part of the bourbon-loving Jeff Douglas, the comic relief, the often drunk, always sardonic sidekick to Tommy Albright, the romantic lead. My role delivered all the funny lines, the best double-entendres. At one point I would show up on stage in plaid kilt, dress shoes, and ankle socks, my skinny legs two sticks to the floor. At the very end, I would be the only one on stage as the curtain came down. Jeff Douglas was a no-brainer part, a guaranteed standing ovation.

Except that every day in rehearsal I was blowing my last line, right ahead of my last exit in the next-to-last scene. In it, Tommy and Jeff have returned from Brigadoon and are holed up in a New York bar. Tommy is desperate to go back to his Fiona. Jeff, well, he's rather unpleasantly drunk, cracking wise, holding a hilarious conversation with himself as counterpoint to Tommy's love-struck yearnings. Jeff's final zinger on the way out the door is designed to bring down the house.

> JEFF: *Put it on my bill, Frank.*
> BARTENDER: *The bill, sir, is very high.*
> JEFF: *So am I!*

Three words for one last laugh—especially when delivered to a high school audience—before the tear-jerker ending. But not when I poured them out as flat as a day-old gin fizz, right up and through dress rehearsal.

Meanwhile, Bill Samuelson was also Jeff Douglas in Sister Regina's double-cast extravaganza. Bill was a senior, maybe 6-foot-3, 240 pounds, a football player on his way to West Virginia University. I hated him. He had nailed the exit line weeks before, and every time it got a big laugh from castmates who had been hearing it forever. They actually made sure to watch when the bar scene was being rehearsed. Then I'd get up there after Bill, boot the line, and everyone would politely look away. Bill tried to help. In truth, he was a good guy. *Put the emphasis HERE,* he'd say. But what's the secret of comedy? Timing. You can or you can't. Bill could. During the senior-class show on Thursday he delivered raucous, foot-stomping laughter.

Friday came my turn, with the junior class in attendance. I was off and running with the first crack. And I was hilarious in my kilt. But I knew I would be only as good as my last three words—and they were out there, lurking. The final bar scene played perfectly—Tommy pining, Jeff whining. I got up to leave, walked across the stage, turned around, and fired back: "So am I!" Then it was exit me, stage left. Before I had disappeared behind the curtain, the audience was howling, clapping, going absolutely crazy. Somehow I had delivered the goods. Backstage I thrust my hands over my head in pure, unalloyed exaltation. Freshman year I broke my arm the third day of football practice. Sophomore year I got cut in the first round of basketball tryouts. My Olympic track dream this year was already fading. So this was, right now, the single greatest accomplishment of my life. I was utterly, completely alive. Enter now Mary Liz.

High school musicals are a boiling cauldron of out-of-control teen angst, teen hormones, teen frenzy. It is amazing that even one of them anywhere in the country ever makes it to opening night. There is a crackling, pervasive tension inherent in putting yourself on stage, maybe for the first time, surrounded by a bunch of kids attempting the same thing, everyone desperate not to look the fool. Marry this vulnerability to a burgeoning confidence, put this sudden sense of a vibrating self in a backstage area that's too dark and filled with too many hidden corners for the adults to keep track of, and you have, quite simply, entered make-out heaven.

I had no desire to bring my arms down to earth. I stood wishing the applause would never end. Everyone should hear that sound once in a life. It was all of an instant, but before it was over Mary Liz, a townsfolk dancer, ran up to me, threw her arms around my shoulders, and kissed me on the neck. It wasn't exactly an official backstage, behind-the-curtain tongue session, but still. Before the applause—my applause become our applause—had finally, finally, finally ended, I was head over heels. Twenty seconds before, Mary Liz had been a junior girl I had probably never noticed; she had meant nothing. Now she was everything. At sixteen, it happens that quick.

Of course, I didn't then ask her out. Nor did I enlist a go-between to talk to her, or even to talk to someone else to talk to her. It was safer to worship from afar. I learned her schedule, so between classes, as a thousand-plus York Catholic baby boomers swarmed the halls, I could happen around a corner and maybe she'd be there for a "Hey, Liz!" If there was a "Hey!" back, the rest of the day unfolded in a blissful, perfect haze.

Once school got out for the year I was off to Lake Skaneateles, one of the New York Finger Lakes, from June through August. Dad's last summer and we didn't go camping. He was fifty now, Mom almost. Maybe they had spent enough nights in sleeping bags. We rented a cabin for six weeks with the Philbins, with the Leahys and Schmitts up for a week or two, plus other York Crowd families—the Mastersons and Andersons—up on some weekends. Dad came up on the weekends as well, and then did his two weeks' vacation during his regular August postinventory escape. It wasn't camping, but Skaneateles (commonly pronounced "skinny-atlas") I remember as a time out of time, blissful and serene.

Early on, Neil Armstrong and Buzz Aldrin took their leaps for mankind. We watched on a tiny black-and-white TV, the antenna just so, our picture more lined and even grainier than what the rest of the world was seeing. No matter. In eighth grade I had fashioned a handmade balsa-wood model of the *Gemini* spacecraft, the two-astronaut precursor to the three-man *Apollo*. I designed it from scratch, eyeballing pictures from *LIFE* magazine as blueprints. It had taken me months. So four years later I was still enough of a space geek when the *Eagle* landed to want to follow the flight from the edge of my seat.

Skaneateles also meant I didn't see Mary Liz again until school started in September. It was too early in the year to have memorized her schedule, so I had to make do with honest-to-goodness, by-accident encounters, few and far between. Not until the end-of-summer/first-week-of-school dance at Wisehaven, the local East York swim club, would I have a chance to, well, I had no idea. But whatever it was, she would have to be there.

She was. In a pale, pale purple sleeveless sweater that was merely beyond imagining, the way it looked on her, and a pastel skirt with a tiny flowered pattern. I situated myself as close to her and her girlfriends as I dared—not so close as to be obvious, not so far as to render it a useless endeavor. Hands in my pockets, I stood there attempting to look ridiculously casual, my heart meanwhile pounding in my throat.

And then she called my name. "Steve," she said, motioning with her arm for me to come over. "You're a good dancer, come on!" I am, actually. My sister had taught me. I like to surprise people: a 6-foot-8-inch white guy who can dance. Either that or I can't and I'm making a complete fool of myself and I don't know it. Like my performance in *Brigadoon*—was I really any good? Who knows? But I got my standing ovation. Now Mary Liz had declared me a good dancer. She was dancing with a girlfriend; I moved in on her. The rest is history.

The dance in September 1969 in York, Pennsylvania, was "The Horse," a driving instrumental by Cliff Noble & Co. It had come out the year before, but once the local live bands got it down, it remained a favorite. "The Horse" featured blaring horns and an up-and-down cadence that perfectly conjured a horse on the gallop. With arms outstretched, curled fingers holding the reins, you bobbed to the music—riding the horse—kicking a foot out in front of you on the downbeat while twisting your hands in the opposite direction. That was it.

Between dances Mary Liz talked with her girlfriends while I stood there politely, fairly transfixed, waiting for the next song to start. Eventually there came a slow dance. The crucial moment had arrived. If Mary Liz and I danced now, we would likely spend the rest of this Wisehaven evening together. I can explain the rules of this no better than I can how some kids get designated cool while others don't. But it was time to take her right hand in my left, slide my right arm around her waist, place my hand on the small of her back. She didn't object. We inched together. I dipped a bit with my right hip, and in the next instant I, Steve McKee, was slow dancing with Mary Liz.

The softness of her! In contrast to me. Her breasts beneath her purple blouse pressed against my chest, just so. Her skirted thigh brushed my pant leg. When she put her head on my shoulder, I resolved immediately to ask her to the homecoming dance next month. Not now immediately, but when the time was right, at the perfect moment. This wasn't it, because . . . it wasn't. And by Tuesday, September 30, 1969, such a moment hadn't revealed itself, either. How could it have, when I'd spent most of the intervening weeks ignoring her?

Yet here she was now on Wednesday, coming to see me unasked.

———————

In *Brigadoon*, the village in the highlands of Scotland appears only once in a lifetime. I know this. The show was in early spring my junior year. Beginning that January I lived at York Catholic. A high school musical is by every definition a *production*; it takes forever to get one up and running. I got to school before 8:00 A.M. My last class ended at 3:00 P.M., and by 3:30 I was on the athletic field for track practice. That was also the year of my Olympic sprint dream. Practice ended about 6:00, and after a quick shower I dashed to the drug store down past the Memorial Ice Skating Rink for an egg-salad sandwich on white bread, potato chips, pickle, and chocolate milkshake.

There's a diet! At 7:00 it was back to the school auditorium for rehearsal until maybe 11:00 P.M. Homework got squeezed in wherever. Weekends were all rehearsal. I saw Mom and Dad maybe ten minutes a day, at breakfast.

So on Saturday night when I finally got back to the house after that evening's public performance (my last; as the senior, Bill Samuelson got the premier Sunday closer), it was as if I were meeting my parents for the first time. Mom and Dad had come to the show that night, of course. With them were a couple of their York Crowd friends. I don't remember who. But they were at the house, some of them, as they all would be five months later. You could depend on the York Crowd, in good times and bad. This was a good time.

I bounded up the five stairs from the foyer to the living room and into one more standing ovation, private and special. At the top stair waited Dad, right hand extended. I will never forget the look on his face when our eyes met. Who was this boy he had seen on stage? Where had he come from? That was part of it. But so too was this: That he recognized exactly who I was, always had, and that he knew someday he'd have reason to be this proud. I reached for his hand. I don't recall that we spoke. Dad's eyes were a brilliant, cut-glass green, and they talked for us.

Ever since, I have taken those eyes everywhere with me. Jeff Douglas is the only real accomplishment I got to share with Dad, in that moment when I was beginning to knock around inside the adult I was becoming, the man he had helped create. Everything else—high school and college graduations, Noreen, my wedding, Patrick, the *Wall Street Journal*,

Alaska, books, everything—they all occurred without him there to see me, look at me. So I remember that night and those eyes, once in a lifetime.

When he died, Dad left no unfinished business between us, so far as it went. We had sixteen years. What he left undone, or left not done, was the rest of my life with him. This realization can come upon me in both expected and unexpected ways. When I was playing basketball for the Centaurs of Allentown College of St. Francis de Sales, Mom made it to most of my games, home and away. If she was late arriving, she made sure to let go with an extra loud "Let's go, Allentown!" when she got to the gym. I wanted to hear Dad's voice, too. Noreen and I married nearly nine years after September 30. The night before, back at Stanford Drive after the rehearsal dinner, I lay on my bed and I cried. My room still looked much as it had when I was in high school, when I started tacking every possible memento from every possible moment to the walls and, eventually, ceiling. The *Brigadoon* program was up there somewhere, I'm sure. Tomorrow he should be here. This went beyond anger. It was pure lament for a life together missed. Or put it this way, unglamorously. A friend told me once that he knew he finally had a complete life with his father when he bumped into him at a strip club. *What are you doing here? What are YOU doing here?* I can't imagine Dad at a strip club. It's been quite awhile for me, too. But I understood exactly what my friend meant.

So without a life together forward, one looks back. I wonder often if everything else being equal, this would be so important to me. If I were sixteen and he were fifty when he died, but the end had come in a car crash, some protracted illness, any way but the way it did—sudden, complete, terrifying, just him and me at home that night—if all this would be necessary. Or if everything had occurred just as it did, but I hadn't been there to witness it. I can't know, of course. So I look back, searching for him in details.

He could walk the fields all day in the fall, hunting pheasant. So there was a time when he was in shape. Or maybe it was just that he was younger then. Once, we were out in the driveway shoveling snow. I was maybe eight, nine years old, making Dad forty, forty-one. When he finished up he came over to where I was playing and told me to hop on his shovel, one of those scooped, plow-like things. I sat down. "Hold on," he said. I grabbed the wood handle and with that he took off running down the street, which was still covered in a hard layer of snow. He sprinted past four or five houses to where Wilshire Drive started up the hill, but instead of stopping he ran himself in a wide circle and brought me around crack-the-whip style and started back up the street. From my vantage point behind him he was silhouetted in the dark, the steam trailing from his mouth like a locomotive's, brightened by the street lamps, his boots chugging on the snow crust. Dad, indestructible.

All of Dad's facts-of-life talks took place in his car. If automobiles have a new-car smell, they can have an old-car smell, too, at least the old jalopies could, like Dad's pale green late-1940s junker. For me, dust, grease, and some worn-out fabric upholstery warmed by a car heater stuck on "high" conjures words like penis and erection, vagina and insertion. Thankfully to-

day's new cars don't smell like that when they age out; I don't
need the mnemonic device. But I can still hear Dad running
through the required vocabulary, and as a father now I appreciate the setting—captive audience, no eye contact. I have employed it myself, passed along his aphorisms. "Never look in a
woman's purse," he told me. "A guy chases a girl until she
catches him." I doubt if that was original to him, but this may
be: "A girl can run faster with her skirt up than a guy can with
his pants down."

He took me for my first driving lesson. He drove the car to the
parking lot at Standard Register. We exchanged places, and
then for probably the next twenty minutes we sat there as he
talked, explaining everything about everything on the dash-
board. Then he had me drive around the lot—in circles, stopping, backing up, straight lines, turns. Then we exchanged
seats and he drove home. Mom took me out the next time. We
skipped the parking lot and went right onto the streets of
Haines Acres, but still inside our neighborhood. "Take it out
on Haines Road," she said. Haines was the main drag, requir-
ing a nasty left turn from Raleigh Drive. That turned onto
Mount Rose Avenue, and the next thing I knew Mom was
telling me to hit the on-ramp for Route 83, the four-lane inter-
state that cut through East York in the 1950s. I have always
considered those two driving lessons as emblematic of the difference between Mom and Dad. I drive like Dad.

He reveled in the longstanding East York price wars between
the Esso gas station at the corner of East Market and Mount

Zion Road and the Workingman's Friend farther down. Workingman's was off-brand—it sold oil in glass jars at 10 cents a quart. Dad bought his oil there, his gas wherever the price was lower, but he always admired the little guy's pluck, taking on the giant company. He'd come home from work and after his whistled greeting announce the day's price: twenty-one-point-nine cents a gallon! 20.9 a gallon! 19.9! When Workingman's dropped to 9.9 cents a gallon, daring Esso to match it, Dad was thrilled.

He could swear, yes. But his favorite oath, employed only occasionally and only for special effect, was the first stanza of The Lord's Prayer, performed with ever-rising incredulity. "Our Father, who art in heaven, hallowed be Thy name!" Except he said it in Greek, the last vestige of his five years in Buffalo's Little Seminary. This attestation had the added benefit of being applicable to any situation, happy or sad, in anger or in joy. I asked a priest at our church for a phonetic spelling, and when he said it at speed it sounded very familiar: *PA-ter hey-MOAN haw en toys oo-ra-noys, ha-gi-as-THAY-tow taw AW-no-ma-sue!*

He infuriated Mom the way he bought her Christmas present. In a good way. He worked on Christmas Eve, of course, not leaving until 3:30, even 4:00 or later. Then it was off to a department store for a quick buy and a gift wrap. He always found the perfect gift, Mom says, and not just in retrospect. It drove her crazy, even as she loved it. Gold-print lounging pajamas she wore for years; hurricane lamps on early-American wooden wall stands; a turquoise birthstone ring. Christmas at our house was a double big deal because Mom's birthday was Christmas Eve. Dad took us to dinner that night, to keep the birthday from getting lost in the season. He made it a huge event—a bag of gifts, a surprise cake, "I'll Never Smile Again." The best restaurant, too: the Flamingo, Hap Miller's, maybe the Jolly Coppersmith up Route 83. Invariably, it seems now, the maître d' was "Mr. Anthony," as he was known in the newspaper ads (locals couldn't pronounce his last name). In 1960, some area doctors and lawyers recruited him from the Black Angus restaurant on Philadelphia's Main Line. He is largely responsible for introducing fine dining and both French and Italian cuisine to York County's Pennsylvania Dutch Country. There was no Caesar salad until Mr. Anthony arrived. (His secret: "A coddled egg—warmed up but still loose. It held the dressing together.") And he prepared his flaming-sword shish kebabs right there at the table. ("It was easy, but everybody'd clap," he says with a laugh.) His daughter went to York Catholic and was a friend of Kathy's. On July 8, 1978, I became Tony D'Ottavio's son-in-law when Noreen married me.

He was a bed wetter, Dad was, at least that's what he told me when I turned out to be one, too. I was probably a freshman in high school before it finally ended. Thinking about it even now I feel rising in me all the latent perturbations of a thirteen-year-old kid trying to stay awake through the night at a sleepover to avoid soaking someone else's bed. For years—and I mean years—Dad got himself up in the middle of the night to get me up to go to the bathroom so I wouldn't pee the bed. It never worked, but he never stopped. It is as vivid a memory as I have of him. I am four, five years old, and after being led to the bathroom I am standing in front of the toilet, eyes closed, all but asleep, my bare bottom nestled against the warmth of Dad's legs as he holds me up to keep me from swaying too much so I don't miss. Camping trips were particularly awful. Dad was convinced the problem was the cold, so he went to great lengths every night to wrap my sleeping bed in a canvas tarp, a 360-degree envelopment. I see him hard at work tucking me in, his face close to mine, his expression saying this time, this night it will work, and you and me will be done with it for good. Then the next morning he would get my bag out and throw it over a line he had strung between two trees so it could air out as long as possible before tucking me in again. He never, ever, got angry at me, lost his temper, ran out of patience.

He had a "great sensitivity," Mom says. Not just that he himself was sensitive, but that he was sensitive to other people's sensitivities. Witness me, the bed wetter. This had to have worked both for and against him. It was surely a button that some of his bosses at Cole Steel knew to push. But it was also the very best of him, too. One York Crowd family had a son with a serious medical situation. His diet needed to be carefully monitored. Once at a restaurant he started crying because he couldn't have ice cream. Olives and peanuts, on the other hand, he liked and could eat. Dad excused himself, went to a store, and came back with a bottle of olives.

He served as Confirmation sponsor for Jimmy Schmitt, the oldest son of Mr. and Mrs. Schmitt. Jimmy was in my grade at school. Dad often took him with us when we went hunting and fishing. Jim is an optometrist. He lives now in upstate Pennsylvania, not far from Little Pine and Worlds End State Parks, the hunter and fisherman I never became. He has trained pointers, the kind of hunting dog Dad kept. He has a forty-acre hunting camp up in New York. When I contacted Jim to ask if he could provide me some remembrances of Dad for this book, he replied in writing: "Your father was one of the most influential people ever in my life."

He taught me well. If Dad was the dutiful son, so was I. Still am. I was never the hellion. I left that to Kathy, watched, and learned her hard lessons as she went toe-to-toe with Dad, and even more so Mom. Once Dad was gone, my deal was sealed. I would do nothing to upset Mom. Nothing, ever. A promise I made to myself, one I swore to consciously. Be home at 11:00? At 10:45 I was through the door. I was preprimed for this responsibility by Dad. Good example: It is the Saturday before the second Sunday in May my junior year. I am at a friend's house. This guy had a genius for organizing the kids who orbited far from the sun of York Catholic High School into their own cohesive group of parallel cool. (That I was at his house is perhaps a more objective indicator than my own opinion of my actual status at YC.) I was not drinking. Of course I was not drinking. Though I don't remember that anyone was, either. It was getting late, and suddenly there was a movement afoot to turn the party into a sleepover. But I knew I couldn't make the call to ask permission. I knew I had to go home. I had to wake up at the house Sunday morning. I had to be home because I knew I couldn't bear the look on Dad's face if I walked in the door sometime tomorrow afternoon. *Didn't you know it was Mother's Day?*

He was a Civil War buff. Not to the level of a re-enactor, but he was a regular reader of Bruce Catton and Shelby Foote, their hardbound volumes on a bookshelf in Mom and Dad's bedroom. Catton's *Terrible Swift Sword* remains one of my all-time favorite book titles. And for years, it seemed, Dad kept a copy of John Pullen's book about the Twentieth Maine Regiment on the end table next to his TV-watching seat on the sofa. Joshua Chamberlain and the Twentieth Maine famously fought at Little Round Top during the Battle of Gettysburg, the encounter that, some say, changed not just the battle or the war but history itself. That Dad ended up living in York, Pa., not thirty miles east of Gettysburg was a godsend. We were always going to Gettysburg. When I took Patrick to the battlefield a good thirty-five years since I had last visited the park, I was stunned by how much of it I recognized precisely. At Little Round Top I walked onto the rock outcropping overlooking the second day's battle. The view is amazing, the realization of what transpired there nearly overwhelming. I stood and did exactly what I'd

watched Dad do many times. I put my right arm straight out in
front of me, my left directly out to my side, shoulder high.
Then with my left I slowly closed off the angle formed by my
arms, getting my bearings on the audacious bayonet charge
that Chamberlain had ordered down the hill after the Fifteenth
Alabama Infantry seemed certain to overrun his far left flank.

Dad was at his best when Judy Ochs came to our house for
Sunday night dinner. Roast beef, mashed potatoes, and gravy.
Judy was Kathy's best friend. Dad adored her. So did I. And
not just because I was the younger brother and Judy was three
years older, a varsity cheerleader dating the vice president of
the school. There was something about Judy that unloosed the
best in Dad, the silly Dad, the relaxed Dad. As the years
moved beyond 1963 and Dad's first heart attack, we saw less
and less of that Dad, but he always appeared when Judy came
for dinner. Who knows why? It doesn't matter; I remain grateful to her. When Judy came to dinner, Dad became the Dad
Mom used to talk about—the "old" Dad, the "young" Dad—
the one who reminded her of Ray Bolger. Not the *Wizard of
Oz* scarecrow, but the pliable, loose-limbed Ray Bolger with
bug eyes and nose too big for his face off on another goofy
dance with Judy Garland in *The Harvey Girls*.

———

Late on an August night in 1989, I sat on the second-story
porch of a vacation house in Ocean City, New Jersey, and
watched a total eclipse of the moon. Slowly, almost impercepti-
bly, it disappeared as if it were slipping through a thin vertical

space between tightly drawn black curtains. It went away by degrees as a rounded darkness slowly overtook its face from right to left. A bit less than two hours later it returned, the process reversing until the entire orb had re-emerged as if through a second slit in the curtains.

I understood exactly what was happening. The earth had come between the sun and the moon, throwing the earth's shadow directly over the lunar face. Astrology, physics, geometry, mathematics—all of humanity's intelligent pursuits were at work here. Yet none of it could explain how I felt in that moment, watching it fold and then unfold. The moon was disappearing! What must it have been like for the ancients when they witnessed the same thing, without benefit of knowing, really knowing, what their eyes were telling them? Even more, seeing it myself, I appreciated their amazement. Yes, the moon, it's disappearing!

For me and the human heart, it has long been very much like that—this knowing but not knowing. Some months after Dad's first heart attack, once he was back at Cole Steel and life was "normal" again, I asked Mom what had happened to Dad. There followed a lesson in the heart, of valves and chambers and ventricles, of electrical impulses and pumping corpuscles. Then Mom said Dad's blood was too thick to get through the blood vessels in his own heart, and that's why it had attacked him. I was ten years old, in the fifth grade. All that blood sloshing around in there, and none of it getting to the heart? A first lesson in irony.

I know more now, of course. I understand. Then again . . . that the action of the heart kick-starts in the sinoatrial node in the right atrium with an electrical impulse—that still amazes me. The word "coronary" itself derives from the Latin word *corona* and the Greek word *koron* because the arteries that surround the heart are said to resemble a crown. But frankly, I don't see it (it's upside down, for one thing). To me it's more like a spider's web or, prosaically, like the roots of a tree that have grown around a misshapen rock and are now clinging to it for dear life. In any event, I remain content to know but not know. Knowledge is everything, yes; but it changes nothing. I once interviewed a comedian, a regular at a Greenwich Village club in Manhattan. He chastised me right off for even attempting to figure out the humor thing. It's like when you dissected the frogs in high school, he said. You know all about it when you're done, but now the frog is dead.

I have grown over time to consider the human heart—or, more accurately, the specific fist-sized, twelve-ounce-or-so, four-chambered, spider-webbed organ pulsing within me—as a living, breathing entity quite apart from the rest of me. It has a personality, a life of its own. I can stand at a remove from my own self and look upon it. When I do, I see both a loyal friend and a distrusted enemy. It doesn't just beat in my chest—*lub-dub, lub-dub*. It talks to me—*LUB-dub, LUB-dub*. It speaks to me, continually reminding me of its presence, asking—no, demanding—that I attend to it. I listen and talk back. You bet I do. Years ago I made my deal with this devil: I keep you in shape, you don't attack me. We have been in long conversation ever since.

As for Dad, I have no idea. He never talked to me about any of this. About his father. About his first heart attack in 1963. About how that first attack affected him, changed him, scared him. I was after all only ten years old. Only very recently, for instance, did I learn that Dad likely had a heart attack (or at the very least some coronary "incident") two, maybe three weekends before the one that killed him. He was fishing Conewago Creek at the YWCA's Camp Cann-Edi-On with Mr. Ochs, Judy's father, who told me the following story.

It was time to leave. Mr. Ochs got himself out of the stream and to the bank when he heard from out in the water Dad calling to him: "I don't think I can get out." By now it was near dark, Dad's voice a disembodied plaint over the water. "I could hear him panting," Mr. Ochs said. "I told him to find a rock and sit down for a while, to rest." Dad did, and there the two of them sat—Mr. Ochs on the bank, Dad out in the Conewago, sixty, seventy yards—until it was good and black. Finally, here came Dad, struggling through the water, breathing hard. He sat down on the bank. "I don't think I can make it," Dad said, looking up the hill to where the car was parked. Mr. Ochs is not a large man. He in fact is short, wiry, irascible, a real character. Dad was a good 6-foot-1, 190 pounds. "I had no idea what I was going to do," Mr. Ochs said to me. "I figured it had to be a heart attack."

Finally, they started up the hill, Dad in front, Mr. Ochs behind, pushing. It was slow going, but they made it. Though once at the car it took Dad another long while to get situated. Then Mr. Ochs went down the hill to collect the gear. "When I got back to the car, your dad was sitting there smoking a cigarette," Mr. Ochs said. They liked to stop for a sandwich and a beer on the way back, but Dad told Mr. Ochs he wanted to get home. "That's when I knew it must be bad," Mr. Ochs said.

Mom knew none of this until I told her; neither did Kathy. Dad just didn't talk about any of it. I have talked with all of Mom and Dad's friends from those days; Dad didn't speak of it to them, either. He didn't even speak of it again to Mr. Ochs. So I wonder all the more what he would have said, had he said it.

I asked Mom if she could explain what Dad was like after his first heart attack. How it changed him, if it changed him, from the man she knew before to the man she was then with after. She didn't answer immediately. Instead, she tapped on her chest and looked past me, trying to find the correct words. "He was," she finally said, and then she stopped talking but kept tapping. "He wasn't introspective," she continued. "He wasn't withdrawn." She was still tapping, and then I could tell she had found exactly how she wanted to say it. "He was 'inner directed' after that first heart attack." That confirmed what I had long suspected and have pieced together with available bits of evidence. That Dad was different after that first heart attack.

A coronary infarction kills heart muscle. Myocardium dies and does not come back. Dad didn't come back, either. I see that now. He could stew, no doubt about it. It was the flip side of that great sensitivity. Mom talks of Dad spending a lot of time in the basement on Wilshire Drive in the first year or so after his heart attack, sitting by himself, drinking a couple of beers. In the basement that had to be finished for him by the guys at Cole Steel. Two or three Black Label beers was all he'd have, but there he'd sit, just . . . sitting. Not reading, which he loved to do, not watching TV, which he also loved to do. "He was depressed," Noreen said upon hearing this later, making a quick and likely correct diagnosis. We know that now. Many of the people who have had a heart attack confront the symptoms of depression in the aftermath. Of course they do. For many of these people it's a major situation. And the depression itself can become its own risk factor.

Kathy and I, when talking of Dad, sometimes start the conversation with one or the other of us saying, "Our father . . . ," with the other, not missing a beat, responding, " . . . who art in heaven!" I don't remember the context or what we were talking about, but one time Mom suddenly brought us up short when she blurted out, "Your father was no saint!" There followed a pause, and then all three of us burst out laughing, her declaration releasing something in all of us, maybe forever, allowing us to consider Dad for what he was—a person, just a person. There was freedom in that.

Dad took his belt to me on very few occasions, almost always the result of another horrible report card. One from fifth grade I still remember: "Unsatisfactory" in conduct; "unsatisfactory" in effort. It was the effort mark that got me the strap. He otherwise never hit me. Except once. I was in sixth grade. Mom had that day received in the mail a picture of her mother taken when Agnes Bunce was four years old. Just recently discovered, it was a rare find for the Famous O'Neil Sisters. The faded brown photo was on hard, brittle cardboard, and Mom told me to make sure not to bend it. So I had to, to see how far it could go without breaking, as soon as she left the room. Not much, as it turned out. It snapped like a stale potato chip right across the middle under the barest of pressure. I taped it back together and sort of half hid it on my dresser. That night as I was getting out of the tub Mom opened the door, photo in hand, absolute hurt across her face. *How could you?* I told her it was an accident. She closed the door. When it opened again there stood Dad, in a complete rage, coming right at me. He slapped me around, five, six, seven times, screaming and yelling, then finished me with a hard right to the chin that knocked me back into the tub, and walked out.

I liked to eat cereal before going to bed. Team Flakes. I was forever leaving the milk out on the counter, which Dad usually discovered the next morning when he came down to the kitchen. One night I was in bed asleep when suddenly there was Dad storming through the door. Before I could move he was over me, pouring the carton of milk on my head. "Maybe that'll teach ya," he said, or something, and clumped out. I sat on the edge of the bed for hours, stunned, the milk drying to a crust in my hair. Mom came in at one point, but I chased her out. I never went back to sleep, and when the sun came up—this was summer, so it was early—I was dressed and packed, with sleeping bag. I was running away. I filled a bag with food, those Team Flakes, undoubtedly, and headed out. I would sleep over in a new section of Haines Acres where new houses were going to be built but for now was still a series of empty lots. I'd spend my days out at the Wisehaven pool. I'd show him. I arrived at my campground and spread out my bag, crawled in, and fell asleep right off. For probably about eight minutes. When I woke up I gathered my stuff and walked home, not in triumph exactly but feeling I had made my point, somehow. Mom and Dad were still asleep. I put everything away and crawled back into bed on the side not newly pasteurized.

In February 1968, Mom threw a surprise five-years-after party to celebrate Dad's clean bill of health from his heart attack in February 1963. Such was the medical wisdom then: Get to five years and you were good to go. Former President Dwight Eisenhower was already at nearly thirteen with his! It was a great time, this party, the York Crowd in top form. Mr. Masterson remembers nearly throwing out his back sneaking the keg into the basement. A surprise party is only as good as its first moment. For this one everyone paraded through the foyer on Stanford, one after the other, with Dad standing on the first step to the living room. He looked stunned, but with that delightfully bemused little smile of his playing with his face. But as a rule, the Februarys after Dad's first heart attack were not good months for us McKees. Mom and Dad did not often fight. I remember one; Kathy remembers one. Both happened in February, in postattack years. Mine came about after Dad said he was going out to get a six-pack on a Saturday night and Mom said that maybe he'd already had enough beer for one weekend after a Friday night party. The three of us were standing in the foyer. He looked at me and then huffed out of the house and didn't come back until Monday. Kathy's also happened in the foyer. This one was more physical, Mom and Dad arguing, with Dad pinning Mom behind the bathroom door for a moment before, again, heading out. Kathy doesn't remember the why of the fight, just that it happened.

Aside from Dad's first heart attack, there was one other time when I felt the tectonic plates shift beneath me. We were still on Wilshire Drive. I came home from school and Dad was home, frantically, bizarrely packing up his brown-and-tan Chevy Fleetwood station wagon, the 1959 model with the huge fins that started at the front door and ran the length of the car. You could sit on them out toward the back, they were so wide. By the time Dad drove away he had it loaded to the gills—suits, shirts, shoes, shotgun, fly rod, waders, everything he owned. The next day Kathy and I were with Mom in our other Chevy, the '63 Biscayne. Suddenly Mom said, "Well, I guess I should tell you what's going on here." Pause. "Dad is afraid he is going to lose his job. He's hitting the road to check on customers." It made perfect sense. It made no sense at all. A couple of days later, no more than two or three, Dad was back. He unpacked the car and we never spoke of it again.

He had anger in him. This went beyond any yearning he may have harbored for the forest ranger's job that couldn't happen, an Australia not returned to, any of that. I can't with any accuracy say how much may have been triggered by that first attack. But when I put the punch in the bathtub, the two fights with Mom, the milk, his pack-the-car disappearance all in a row, knowing that they took place between the attack that felled him and the one that killed him, I can't help but think it was more than a little.

I have come to understand his anger, in the same way I now understand the yearning that got me to Alaska. I spent years being angry, quietly, softly angry, just like him. I spent more years in therapy talking about it, and if I hadn't found some peace with it I likely would have lost Noreen, thereby losing it all. The precipitating moment? In May of 1995 a pair of utility workers came to our door asking if they could check our tenant's meter downstairs. When it seemed to be taking more time than it should, I wound my way down the spiraling stairs, absentmindedly picking up a hammer on the steps along the way. This basement was something out of an Alfred Hitchcock movie, dark and crowded. I stopped at the door and asked what they were doing. Looking to shut off the electricity, they said. At which point I lost it, completely lost it, yelling and screaming—while holding the hammer by the claw. After more yelling and screaming the utility people left. The next day, two police detectives knocked on my door.

I was forty-three and a half years old. Six months from the age when Dad had his first heart attack. It would be incorrect and misleading to figure that my being this age and the cops at my door was a simple A-equals-B calculation. But it got my attention, anyway. All of this got my attention. I decided not to cling to the fact that the utility people had gotten into the basement under false pretenses. Or that they weren't supposed to be there. Or that I had made no motion toward the utility workers and that I had put the hammer down as soon as it registered that I had it in my hand. No, this rage of mine had brought two police detectives to my front porch. I had spent too many of my growing-up years with a father who could stew, who was quietly, softly angry. That's how I saw it; how I knew I needed to see it. I had learned too well. This was some of the Dad I did not want to become; in fact, what I was here went far beyond the Dad I didn't want to become. Kathy actually had the best observation about her perfect younger brother and his dilemma, and she offered it not without some justifiable older-sister delight: "You screwed up. You finally screwed up!"

Mom says she and Dad shared many good times—weeks, months, *years*. And as with any marriage, she says, there were bad times, too, and she could live with that. But now, she says, turn those good and bad times into numbers on a chart, with February 2, 1963, the before-and-after dividing line. For all the good ones before, there would be that many bad ones after. And if there had been only a few bad in all the years prior to February 2, 1963, there were only a few good in the 2,430 days that followed. It was that black and white.

In the early 1980s I asked Mom why she and Dad had had only two children. I remembered her telling me and Kathy that Dad had wanted an even dozen and that while Mom probably wasn't on board for all that, six, seven, eight would have been great by her. At our St. Joe's parish, I can think right off of four families at Sunday Mass with ten-plus kids lined up down the pew, week after week. Nearly all the York Crowd

families were some combination of five, six, or seven. The Mc-
Kee's single pair was clearly an aberration.

They had an active sex life until she was forty, Mom told
me. And they were always hopeful that the next time would be
the time. Post forty, she said, they were more careful, in a Roman Catholic rhythmic sort of way. As to why only two, they
never knew, and neither did the doctors. Mom was nearly
twenty-seven when she married in 1947, and she didn't con-
ceive with Kathy for a full twelve months. In the rush to nor-
malcy of the postwar years, that was cause to worry. Mom
consulted doctors, who declared she would likely never have
children. Then, Kathy, and the doctors told Mom there was no
reason Dad couldn't have his dozen. But it took eighteen more
months just to get me started.

My birthday is November 17, 1952. Give me a minute and I
can name twenty-five, thirty people whom I know personally
with that same date. Four or five kids in grade school, another
five in high school, still more in college, friends of friends, on
and on. I once counted back the required forty weeks and arrived suspiciously close to . . . St. Valentine's Day. I said this to
Mom when we were having our little "talk" about Dad's de-
sired dozen. She immediately said, "Oh, no, that wasn't the
day, it was . . ." That's where I cut her off, my need for information fully sated.

So, years later when I was pressing her on how Dad's first
heart attack had changed him and she started first with her
chest tapping, I wasn't surprised when later she offered unso-
licited that the man with whom she had spent a good nine

years trying for a third kid had "completely lost interest in sex" after that attack. She never learned why. He certainly never told her. Perhaps the doctors ordered him to stop. Maybe Dad just decided he should. There's a bit of death in love done well with the right person. That full surrender. Perhaps Dad had tarried too close to the real thing on February 2, 1963.

In those years between his heart attacks, there was one more incident that took place between Dad and me. It was in my junior year in high school, late February, early March, not more than a few weeks before *Brigadoon,* in fact. I remember because when I ran out of the house it was snowing—big, wet, spring flakes— and there were already a couple of inches on the ground.

Dad and I got into a fight, an actual fists-up, come-and-get-it squaring off. It was a Saturday night. Mom wasn't home; she was away for the weekend, I think at a Catholic women's retreat, which she attended with some regularity. It started with Dad and me goofing around, a pretend slap fight, laughing and joking. Then all of a sudden it wasn't pretend anymore. How it got from one to the other, I haven't a clue. Next thing we had each other by the shirt collars, trying to throw each other off, until he got the upper hand and manhandled me into a chair, an upholstered rocker that spun in circles. It was my favorite chair for TV watching; I liked to throw my leg over one of its padded arms and use my foot to knock it back and forth. I don't know how it didn't break, the way Dad put me down.

The abruptness of that move brought the action to a momentary halt, the two of us still holding each other by the collar.

I broke his grip and stood up. We stared at each other, breathing heavy. Finally I said, "It's a good thing you're my father," trying to imply that were he not, I would have beat the crap out of him right there. I have no idea if I would have, could have, followed through on that threat. Instead I ran upstairs, changed into my running gear, and headed to the front door.

Dad called to me when I got outside. I stood in the snow, waiting for him to come out to me. "I'm sorry," he said once he reached me. I sensed that he wanted to say something else, but I don't recall that he did. Instead, we stood next to each other, the snow collecting in our hair. I started to cry. After a few long seconds I turned and ran down the steep hill of Stanford Drive, the spring storm surrounding me in silence.

I have often wondered what to make of that night—while at the same time cautioning myself not to make too much of it. But I do think this. When I broke Dad's hold and stood up, we weren't looking at each other eye to eye. By then I was probably 6-foot-3, maybe 6-foot-4—a sizable three or four inches taller than Dad. I had overtaken him. In the same way, perhaps, that his life had overtaken him. He was already down one heart attack by age forty-four. Now, he had just turned fifty. He was a smoker, addicted. As for Cole Steel, don't get him started. If Dad gave up after that first attack knocked him over, and he never really got up off the canvas after that, perhaps that night is when he finally stopped trying at all. I have no idea why that night happened the way it did, but I think in some ways it served to pass the baton from him to me. Here, Steve, you take it, I give up. I remember his eyes, again the eyes, as I looked down into them as we went chest to chest in the TV room. Angry and raging, helpless and tired.

———

I asked Mary Liz to the homecoming dance when she came to see me Wednesday night. For all the wrong reasons, I had found the perfect moment. Or, rather, it had found me. Like when I would return to York Catholic on Tuesday a week later, and I discovered because of events I was now orbiting close to the center of the solar system. It wasn't my fault I was there—but I liked it.

She said no. She said she had just been asked that day. I prided myself on taking the high road—that I was head over heels for a girl with the self-esteem and dignity not to break a promise made. Though had she even hinted at a willingness to get out of that first invitation, I would have begged her to tell him no, that she was going with Steve, that his father just died, shameless in pressing my case.

We were now out front of the Schmitt's house on Sundale Drive. Last night, this was the house I had run to from Stanford Drive to get Mom, to tell her Dad was dead. Mary Liz and I were here because right before I had first seen her in the door window at home, Mr. Schmitt had told me he had arranged for his son Jimmy to get a few of the guys together and have me come over. "Don't think you need to stay here," he said. "Don't feel guilty. Relax. Have some fun. We'll take care of your mom." Except now with Mary Liz here there was no place else I wanted to be. A fact Mr. Schmitt surmised quickly; all he had to do was look at me. But the guys were already on their way. He told me and Mary Liz to go get something to eat, take about an hour, and then she could drop me at their house. Go to Gino's, he said.

For those of us who grew up on the east end of York, the original fast-food hamburger chain isn't McDonald's, it's Gino's. In fact, McDonald's had yet to arrive in York by September 1969. No, as Gino's own slogan sang it, "Everybody goes to Gino's! 'Cause Gino's is the place to go!" And here I was, going with Mary Liz. Gino's was owned by Gino Marchetti, the great defensive end for the great Baltimore Colts teams of the 1950s and 1960s, just south into Maryland on Route 83. The Colts were York's team. In the winter months they would sometimes come up to play benefit basketball games. When I was in eighth grade and playing in the C.Y.O., I was on a team that played the preliminary before the Colts took on the "Double Dribblers," the basketball team of the WSBA "Good Guys," the local AM radio station, nine-ten on the dial, the one to listen to before school to know what songs to talk about that day. After our prelim at York Catholic we went to the locker room and there they were: the Colts, with Coach Don Shula making a surprise appearance with the team. Some were taking pregame showers. We eighth graders huddled around each other until the Colts motioned to us to come on in, the water was fine. So we did. This was no small deal. These were the mighty "Bal-mer" Colts. Just a month ago, after all, with both Johnny Unitas and his backup, Gary Cuozzo, hurt, running back Tom Matte had stepped under center as quarterback *with the plays taped to his wrist*. In the last game of the season he led the Colts to a 20–17 win over the Los Angeles Rams to force a one-game playoff with the Green Bay Packers the day after Christmas. The Colts had lost that one, 13–10 in overtime, but we all knew they had been cheated. Don Chandler's kick to tie it for the Pack at the end of regulation was wide right, even if the ref said it wasn't. So yeah, no small deal, this showering with the Colts (impossible as it is even to fathom such a thing today). At the same time this was no big deal at all. They were just the Colts. Sports was different then, and these regular guys in their blue shirts with the white numbers were emblematic of the time. Yeah, Gino's was the place to go.

Though not the perfect place to ask Mary Liz to the dance. Not until we arrived at Schmitts and we were standing next to her car and she had to leave and so did I, did I finally ask her. Honestly? I thought I was a lock. How could she say no? But as she turned me down, she offered hope. The week after homecoming, she said, we'll see a movie—*Funny Girl,* all the dates were going to it—and we'll wear what we wore to the homecoming. I asked another girl to the dance if only to acquire an official homecoming outfit. The theme was "Romeo and Juliet," a homage not to Shakespeare but to the Franco Zefferelli film that had come out the year before and that all of us had seen. Leonard Whiting as Romeo and Olivia Hussey as Juliet, and they were both our age. And there was that bedroom scene—that's why we went—with Romeo bare from behind and Juliet naked to the waist. You could see her, only for an instant, but you could. Yet still the nuns had told us to go!

Walking into the homecoming dance at York Catholic, I was fully one with the drama of a star-crossed, young-lovers romance. Early on, Mary Liz walked over and whispered in my ear that next Friday would be our Friday. And so it was. My suit was one of Dad's gray wool herringbones that Mom took to a tailor to have taken in and made longer. It didn't fit me—the pants revealed two inches of black sock, the jacket was tentlike—but I wore it anyway, hoping the electric-pink shirt and charcoal checked tie would dazzle enough that Mary Liz wouldn't notice.

If she did, she was too polite to say. She looked beautiful, dressed in navy blue, with white stockings. *Funny Girl* was playing downtown on George Street at either the Strand or the Capitol, a pair of fabulously old-fashioned movie houses with marble floors and acres of gold leaf. I wager no one in York knows which is which, even today, unless standing beneath the double marquee. When Omar Sharif came to Barbra Streisand before going to jail and said, "So long, Funny Girl," Mary Liz leaned into me and said, "I'm going to cry now." She couldn't have been more direct had she clicked on a neon sign that read: "Put your arm around me so I can put my head on your shoulder." The movie ended too quickly after that.

I drove her home slowly, not wanting the night to end, but with no idea how to prolong it. At her front door I stood as helpless in her presence as I'd been the night we slow danced at Wisehaven. Any move now was her move. All I could do was wait. She put her arms around my neck, rose on her tiptoes, and kissed me. Long. Well, not long. But it seemed long. Until it was over.

My senior year at York Catholic I wrote lots of bad poetry—I was "Broomstick"; Mary Liz "Tiger"; Dad "Green Eyes." I spent hours driving the York circuit—Philadelphia Street to West York, then back east on Market Street, the main drag. I added my own private spur, past Mary Liz's house, driving fast enough to make it look like I was going somewhere, not so fast that if she happened to be outside she'd have time to wave and then I could pull over. *Hey, just driving by.* I never saw her.

When Mary Liz came to see me that Wednesday night, less than twenty-four hours after Dad died, I didn't know the beginning and end were one and the same. I did walking down her steps that *Funny Girl* night. I was a fool in love, but not an idiot. The guy she went to homecoming with, he was the one. A few years later she even ended up married to him for a while. I never asked her out again. I wanted to, was desperate to. I knew it was useless. But why had she come to see me Wednesday night?

The spring musical was *South Pacific*. It rescued senior year. I was Luther Billis, the no-brain comic relief again, in this one cavorting in a grass skirt and a pair of coconut-shell boobs. Are you kidding? Standing ovation, guaranteed. At a dance the night of the senior show on Friday, I employed my weekend at the top of the Fightin' Irish status chart to ask a girl named Sally, a senior member of the stage crew, to the prom. I'd been tipped by a go-between that she was interested. She was very nice. We had a good time at the prom.

There was another girl, not at York Catholic, but from out at the pool and down at the York Mall. I heard one of the guys say he had copped a feel on her—top and bottom both—and I decided to see if I could too. Turned out I could. It was hurried, joyless, clinical—*so, it feels like that*. Though not so much, I suppose, that I didn't return to her again, a few months later. The Monday after the second encounter I saw her at the mall. I was with friends. We were walking toward each other, and she was obviously trying to get my attention. I didn't let her. I stared past her and kept moving. This girl was a solution that didn't work, that couldn't work, and I wronged her in trying to find it with her. I wanted to be with Mary Liz. Of course, with Mary Liz there would have been none of that. It was all too confusing, the ache within me too piercing to permit understanding.

It wasn't until I went off to college the next September that I got past Mary Liz and the startling fact that she had appeared in the window of the door that Wednesday night. I finally stopped trying to figure out why. It was enough to remember that she had and in doing so how her presence had made all else fall magically, blissfully away. In the one moment when I needed that most. Like Dad in all things, like a total eclipse of the moon, she remains for me another lesson in the workings of the heart.

WEDNESDAY,
OCTOBER 1; 3:00 P.M.

EVENTS WERE HAPPENING NOW ONE ON TOP OF THE OTHER, TOO quickly to keep pace. It was barely the middle of the afternoon, less than a day later, and already my green herringbone suit was off to the cleaners; Mr. Kirk had been dispatched to buy me a black tie; we had been visited by Mr. Keffer of the funeral home; Kathy was back from Buffalo and with her Aunt Evie and Aunt Marg. The three of them came into the house together and everyone started crying, and I realized that's the way it was going to be, and for who knew how long. Whenever I saw someone, I was required to cry. If not for my sake, then theirs.

Now Kathy and I were on our way to West York, to the coffin place. Down Haines Road to East Market, across to Memory Lane and then between the gargantuan Caterpillar complexes that had completely transformed East York in the mid-1950s. I asked Kathy how she'd heard about Dad last night. She said Uncle Leo found her at Brinks, one of the many college hangouts along Elmwood Avenue in Buffalo. Uncle Leo was a city policeman, by then way up the ranks, but he still knew his way around. Now here he was, and for Kathy completely out of context. Walking toward him, Kathy said, everything went into slow motion. *This cannot be good.* "Tell me, just tell me," Kathy said. Your dad had a heart attack. "Is he dead?" Yes. She went back in the bar and sat on the windowsill for a long time.

With Kathy's story told it was my turn. Not for the first time, not for the last, as I was quickly learning. People wanted to hear about last night. For their sake or mine, I never figured out, but they wanted to hear it. Kathy was different. She needed to hear it, and I needed to tell her. Somewhere in this recounting came the song "One" by Three Dog Night on WSBA, 910 on the AM dial.

Music, the songs of the moment that we grow up with, that we heard without hearing, knew without knowing how. If our life were a movie, they would be its soundtrack. This is not an original thought, but it's no less true for not being one. Hear them now and they don't just jar a bit of memory, they transport you back, enveloping you in a particular time, a specific place, a certain emotion.

"When a Man Loves a Woman," by Percy Sledge. Our St. Joseph eighth-grade graduation party—Class of '66!—and much to my relief Joan Galloway has asked me to dance. She and Danny Quinlivan were the first couple in a "snowball," an effort by a WSBA deejay to breathe life into a dying party. Danny and Joan danced, the music stopped, and they each found new partners. Five or six music stops later—plenty of options still available—Joan asked me. At our twentieth reunion I told her this story while we were dancing again. All that was missing was my fifteen-minute erection, though I didn't tell her that.

"Na Na Hey Hey Kiss Him Goodbye," by "Steam." Steam is in quotes because we all knew it wasn't a real band, just three guys who threw a song together at the last minute—the "Na-Nas" being where the words would go had they thought of any, at least that was the story—and then watched it hit No. 1 in December 1969. When I hear it now, I'm playing basketball in college, and the goodbye part serenades me off the floor after fouling out again on the road. Once it would be with a full band right behind our team, trombones jabbing, with me on the bench . . . steaming.

"What's Goin' On?" by Marvin Gaye. I am in college and wondering what next. I want more than a job, more than some nine-to-five and then home for dinner to complain for twenty minutes. But how? Where? What's going on? I haven't a clue.

"Hollywood Swinging," by Kool & the Gang. Twenty-two now, out of college, on my way soon to St. Mary's, Alaska, with the Jesuit Volunteer Corps to teach at a boarding school. But timing is everything, at least sometimes. I am amazed to be dancing with Noreen D'Ottavio, a senior-girl member of the York Catholic homecoming court when I was a freshman. A bit of that amazement is with me still. We are doing "The Bump"—that mid-1970s embarrassment where couples banged hips, shoulders, and elbows, plus assorted other body parts, maybe, perhaps auguring well for later in the car. We have just recently met. She never asks me not to go to Alaska.

"Love Will Lead You Back," by Taylor Dane. I am in a rental car in a small town thousands of miles from Brooklyn.

Noreen and a three-day-old newly adopted Patrick are in the back seat. She and I were in the birthing room when he was born. Our infertility and adoption ordeals had left me ragged, emotionally empty, as if a soup ladle had scraped out every last bit of me. Now here was exactly eight pounds of baby boy replacing my ache with an unspeakable joy, touching me in places vulnerable and exposed where I hadn't dared stray since Dad had died.

Which leads back to "One," by Three Dog Night. I hated it then; I hate it now. But when I hear it on one of those FM oldies stations that has baby boomers like me squarely pegged, it puts me in our blue 1963 Chevy Biscayne, Kathy driving, on our way to pick out a casket for Dad.

———

Kathy and I woke up every morning to the sounds of the same alarm clock: Dad's cough, his cigarette hack. The cilia in Dad's airways, given an overnight reprieve from all that cigarette smoke, were trying now to sweep out some of the gunk that had settled in the lungs in the past few hours. These broomlike hairs never had a chance.

His cough was, in a way, its own musical composition. It had rhythm and cadence and an awful familiarity. There was, first, a raspy breathing-in of air. Then a quick pause, followed by a double exhalation, the first hack longer than the second cough, separated one from the other by a slight catch in the throat. *Breath in. Pause. HACK. (Catch.) Cough.* They came in stanzas—three, four, five at a time, the second-to-last always the highest crescendoed. It was how you knew a particular compo-

sition was about to end. It rendered the final cough a weak impersonation, a faint echo of air oozing from a battered chest.
Then there was silence. No way to say how long. But it would
start again—it always started again—with the sound of his
breathing in, preparing his next arrangement.

He was first up in the morning. For his first cigarette he was
on the toilet. For the second (and probably a third) he was in
front of the mirror, shaving. *Breath in. Pause. HACK. (Catch.)
Cough. "Kathy, Steve. Time to get up."* Mom would be up next
and off to the kitchen, where coffee, cinnamon toast, and fry-
ing eggs were added to the mix, Dad's cigarette smoke always
first among the many. Eventually Kathy would get up, and
with her WSBA radio. Then me last, always last. Ironically, as
much as I hated the cigarettes, as much as I despised the
coughing they induced, conjuring all this back to life is not un-
pleasant. They are the sounds and smells of the McKee family
at 7:15 on a Tuesday morning, circa 1962. I remember too
well.

Dad and cigarettes go hand in hand because Dad always
had one in his. He didn't reek of smoke (dusty, dirty, disgust-
ing); he smelled of tobacco (rich, regal, rewarding). It is a dis-
tinction without a difference, I know, but it is important to me.
Because when I remember Dad, I remember the smokes, and
when I remember them I am desperate for pleasant memory. I
recall he smoked L&Ms, the first of the new filtered brands,
out by 1952. But Kathy says I'm wrong. Prior to his first coronary, she says, Dad smoked Pall Mall unfiltered. She has this
on her own good authority: she started smoking about then
and snuck Dad's to get going. So I defer to her. After the first

attack we agree he turned to Winston, then spent a couple of years with Marlboro and its "Selectrate Filter." Not long before September 30, 1969, he switched to Kool Filter King. The menthol was said to make the cigarette safer.

I have arrived in the writing of this book to the view of Dad as a sort of Everyman of his generation—not its Average Joe, not its Typical Guy, but rather a representative thereof. He wanted nothing more than that, and he achieved it. Carefree kid in the Roaring Twenties. Depression Era teen looking for a job. Young man caught in global events. Eager postwar husband-father-businessman. This Everyman observation extends to his smoking habits, because here Dad was a one-person, unscientific survey on the power of advertising, back when cigarette ads were in magazines, on TV, absolutely everywhere. Pall Mall was the best-selling smoke in America. Winston would eventually take the top spot, and Marlboro was rising with a bullet after Philip Morris finally clicked with its "Marlboro Man" and "Marlboro Country" ad campaigns, riding the theme song from *The Magnificent Seven.* The allure of Marlboro to a man who affectionately called his truck drivers "cowboys" and who himself wished to ride off to Australia and "America's Wild West" I find ineluctable.

It is unclear when Dad started smoking, but the likely culprit is the confluence of World War II, the Army Air Corps, and the millions of cigarettes distributed to American servicemen for a breathing-in of the home front. What a perfect scam that was. His dad, Jack McKee, didn't smoke. In the 1930s, Dad spent the first five of his teenage years in the seminary and the next five, 1938 through 1942, still at home. It is difficult to imagine him walking into Nana's house with cigarette dangling. He may have been by then, but neither Mom nor Dad's sister Alice remembers him smoking before he left for the South Pacific. Once in the service, all bets were likely off. "Know what I'm doing as I write?" Dad typed in a letter to Nana, Mary Jane, and Alice dated September 6, 1944. "I'm smoking a seegar#&%_%. Yup—I'M A MAN NOW. If this letter gets a little hazy you'll know what it is. Doesn't gotoo gab thu. Glub segar. OK, I'll put it down now." In the snapshots we have of Dad from after the war, it is nearly impossible to find one of him without a cigarette in the picture too. (The cover of this book notwithstanding.)

I see him sitting in "his" chair (the left side of the couch, actually) watching TV, reading, smoking, drinking a Coke or maybe a beer, multitasking. As with his cough, I remember this exactly. He reached across his body to get the cigarette from the ashtray with his right hand, put the cigarette in his mouth, and took a drag while reaching for his highball glass with his left. His drag done, he removed the cigarette and took a drink. As he took a swig, he exhaled the smoke through his nose so that it filled up and then overflowed the glass in a billowing cloud that enveloped his face and head and hair before joining the haze that hung in the room. Done, he put the glass on the end table, maybe flicked the end of the cigarette over the ashtray, and readied himself to do it again.

In less than ten seconds his lungs had been filled with hundreds, perhaps thousands of chemicals—rat poison, embalming fluid, nail-polish remover, and car exhaust, to name four possibilities. His alveoli, the tiny, supple air sacs that absorb oxygen deep in the lungs, had been rendered incrementally less pliable, less efficient. His blood vessels had constricted and his heart rate had increased. Most important, his brain had been delivered of its demand for nicotine, and in gratitude rewarded him by releasing pleasure-inducing tonic, the addictive circle closing tighter.

Mom smoked, too, back then. There are pictures of her prewar with cigarette in hand. In one—from 1940, in bathing suit out at the lake, ever the independent—she is nineteen. Mom's two sisters, Marg and Ev, smoked their entire lives, and took the cigarettes with them to the grave (though they did live to eighty-three and seventy-six, respectively). Mom quit for good in 1964, after Dad's first heart attack. "I wanted to show him how easy it was," she says, her voice still combative. Prior to that she had quit a number of times, and for extended periods, but she always picked it up again. Mom's smoking affected me very differently than Dad's. In the earliest years I can remember, it didn't bother me. She obviously smoked way fewer cigarettes than he did, and she smoked Salem, a filtered menthol cigarette, and that had to be better, right? But as I got older and Mom quit more often, seemingly successfully, her smoking came to upset me in a way that Dad's didn't. There was an inevitability to Dad's smoking. It couldn't be defeated. Nothing could be done. But Mom, she could do it; she already had. It got to where when she returned to smoking she would try to hide it from me. It was such an unsettling sight that when I found out she was smoking again it could send me to my bedroom to pull the covers over my head.

Dad did try to quit. He apparently swore off cigarettes while still in the Army Air Corps in the South Pacific. For a short time, at least, his letters home included the marvels of how much better the food tasted and how his cigarette cough had vanished. "I should have quit a long time ago," he declared. Mrs. Leahy tells of a New Year's Eve party—1968, she thinks, Dad's last—when she and Dad and another York Crowd dad resolved to quit. It was beginning to sink in, she says, that maybe they weren't kidding when they said smoking could be bad for your health. "We were at Philbins and we were having our last cigarette at five to midnight," she says. Mrs. Leahy quit for a good ten years. Dad and the other smoker lasted until the next morning and the New Year's Day get-together at our house. "I could have wrung their necks," Mrs. Leahy says with a laugh. I know the feeling, minus the laughter. How many times did Kathy and I come home from school to have Mom collect us up to say, "When your father gets home from work tonight, I want you to be extra good, real quiet, because . . ."? We could finish for her: ". . . because this morning your father gave up smoking." We never had to be extra good more than one night in a row.

Why couldn't he quit? If in those years between his heart attacks I put such stock in his getting out there with me on the junior high track for some exercise, I put even more hope into his giving up the cigarettes. They were the tangible evidence that he was killing himself—one smoke, one pack, one carton at a time. The math was inexorable. Impale Cole Steel as the third point in this triangle and we have the unholy trinity that still haunts me. But cigarettes remain first among equals. Why couldn't he quit? I will never understand.

And I never will, my sister says, because I've never smoked. So I rely on her to guide me here. Kathy started smoking in 1964, when she was fifteen. She quit, finally and for good, in January 1988, at thirty-eight. Twenty-four years of smoke. At the end she was at three packs a day, same as Dad. "That I was able to quit is a complete miracle," she says. There is a story Mom tells of Kathy about three weeks into her quitting for good. How you doing, Kath? Mom asked. Okay, she said, okay. She was going to succeed, she said. She could tell. She would never have a cigarette again. And then she said: "But I know I will never be happy again." That wasn't true, of course, but that's what cigarettes do.

"Smoking was a real good friend of mine," Kathy told me, remembering. Even all these years later it remains easy for her to conjure the smoking life. "You need a cigarette. You're happy, you're sad, you're excited, you're calm. It doesn't matter. With everything you do, you need a cigarette. You sit down. You take a deep breath. You pull out the cigarette. You look at it and start thinking about what you're going to be thinking about when you're smoking." And the ritual begins. "You put it in your mouth. You light the match, put it to the cigarette. You take a drag. And now I'm set. I'm relaxed. I'm in the zone.

"Now, do that sixty times a day," she says.

"Smoking was part of me. I almost miss it just talking about it. Almost." She shrugs. "It was part of Dad. I'm trying to work up some anger for you here, but I can't. I understand him. If he had been able to quit, he would have. The long-term effect of quitting would have been way better, but the immediate effect was so stressful he couldn't even think about doing it. With all this other stuff going on? He hated his job. He'd had a heart attack. Any time he tried to quit, he must have been jumping out of his skin. It is that hard. He had to smoke. He . . . couldn't . . . not . . . do . . . it."

———

With every cigarette Dad smoked, every alarm-clock cough he hacked out, every morning when he didn't get up and head with me down to the junior high track, I promised myself again that I would always keep myself in shape. (That I would never smoke was foregone.) My junior-year dream to become America's next great sprinter was just that, a dream. But I took with me something very concrete from those months of running in the morning, of getting myself up and down to the track. Shape was key. No, for me it was everything.

Back then keeping my stay-in-shape promise was easy. Actually, it was easier than that. I played basketball in college; in the summer I was an every-night regular on York's outdoor courts. For employment I was a playground instructor; for transportation I rode a bicycle (though I originally bought the bike in response to the Arab oil embargo of the early 1970s, with gas topping—what?—forty cents a gallon).

After college, off to Alaska, the guy teachers at St. Mary's played hoops two, three nights a week, full-court four-on-four.

Lots of running—had to stay warm, the cavernous gym was maybe 60 degrees. I learned to cross-country ski, as good a cardiovascular exercise as exists. Post St. Mary's, back in York, I got myself in basketball shape to try out for a lower-division team in France. I failed at that, and Noreen and I were in Fairbanks, Alaska, by September 1978. There, I found something like the basketball I had searched for in Europe. Basketball was invented to get through the winter, and Fairbanks has it. From Halloween to St. Patrick's Day it was all hoops. The University of Alaska–Fairbanks was a very good NAIA school in those days, and many of its players had remained in the city and were sprinkled throughout the upper-division rec league. Tuesdays and Thursdays were league nights; weekends were for tournaments, at the Army base, the Air Force base, the county jail. Competitive games, great runs. The first year I kept track. I played in fifty-four games in about six months; rarely sat out; averaged fifteen points per; once went for forty-four.

The next year it was more of same, with the addition of the Arctic Winter Games, an Olympics-style competition between Alaska and Yukon and Northwest Territories, in Whitehorse, Yukon Territory. I was on the Alaska senior men's team. It was March 1980, less than a month after Lake Placid and the Eric Heiden/"Miracle on Ice" Olympics. That us part-time jocks were now gathered at a let's-pretend Olympics was of no never mind. The Arctic Winter Games became the Quadrennial I had aspired to back on the junior-high track. We slept in a classroom-turned-dormitory at the high school. The real world—the Iran Hostage Crisis; Jimmy Carter's boycott of the

Moscow Summer Olympics—ceased to exist. I played well, rarely coming out of the forty-minute games, and Team Alaska won (in truth, it was a lopsided competition). Our gold medals were shaped like an Eskimo *ulu*, a crescent-shaped knife with a handle in the middle. To cut with an *ulu* you chop straight down with the widest section of the rounded blade, then roll the edge back and forth along its circumference. The Arctic Winter Games were the best five days of my basketball career, such as it ever was.

So being in shape, that was easy. Now fast forward fifteen months, to May 1981. Noreen and I were living and working at the university; I didn't need the bike for summer transportation. I also hadn't played basketball that winter. I'd turned to volleyball; great game, but there were fewer opportunities to play, and not much running. I was still cross-country skiing, but it had all turned very hit-or-miss, my stay-in-shape promise. I just didn't know it. Until in early May when I was hiking the Alaska pipeline corridor north of Fairbanks. With a friend, we were scouting some acreage to be made available by the state in one of its periodic land lotteries.

The terrain was hilly—mountainous by any standard except Alaska's. We were no more than two miles in, not even halfway up the first climb, when I felt my legs leave me, completely disappear. The realization shocked and scared me. I had to stop periodically—checking the map! I said—to catch my breath, pull it together. There I was, hands on my knees, head down, chest heaving, the sweat funneling off the tip of my nose. This wasn't supposed to happen. I had promised it never would. I was stunned.

I had become Dad, or at least a specific remembrance of him. The two of us had once been out walking. Were we camping? Fishing? Just out around the block? I can't say. But we were walking, and it seemed like not every hundred yards we had to stop so Dad could put his hands on his knees, take some deep breaths, get it back together. I stood there, hugely embarrassed—for him, for me. He couldn't even go for a walk.

Now I couldn't walk this hill. I was six and a half months from being twenty-nine years old, but suddenly that was almost thirty. I have no idea if I had any kind of heart "incident" at that moment. It doesn't matter, because I never gave a thought to checking with a doctor anyway. No, I knew immediately what I had to do: get in shape, start running. My focus from the days at the junior high track returned with a resolute clarity.

I had a few times attempted to start running regularly, build a routine. Except for my junior-year Olympic dream, none had ever stuck. Dad called it "road work." Not that he planned to do it himself, but back when I was in grade school and the St. Joe's Black Knight basketball tryouts loomed, he used to tell me it was time for "road work" to get ready for the season. I'd last a day, maybe two, then have to drag myself through the first few practices. Dad came to all my games, but he wasn't the kind of father who hovered at his son's practices—I appreciated that he viewed them as my responsibility—but one time he showed up before an early practice was over to pick me up. I was slogging out our final laps; Dad sitting on the stage by the door at the old York Catholic gym way out on King Street in West York. The place was a furnace, the heating system directly under the foul lane at the far end. The black tiles would get so hot they could be squished around with a sneaker. You did not want to get knocked to the floor under that basket. On one of my laps as I was heading back down to the heat, Dad called out, sotto voce, "Road work!" I did not walk over and smack him in the forehead. For many reasons I fought the urge, not the least of them being that he was right.

Maybe that is why I had never before successfully established a running routine, a fitness regimen, beyond the junior high. Because Dad's "road work" is in fact an apt description of what transpires. This is one of the few things I can say I have learned from a lifetime of staying in shape: It is rarely "fun." That's the great myth of the fitness promise. You can be glad to do it. You can feel good doing it. You can be self-righteously, sanctimoniously satisfied when you're done (for me, a common occurrence). You can even establish it as such an integral part of your life and being that not to do it leaves you bereft, unwhole, and unfinished for the day. Still, it is what it is: work.

Spurred by the memory of Dad sucking wind on a gentle walk, the day after doing the same on that hill in Alaska, I laced up an old pair of high-top Adidas basketball sneakers—the originals with the big rubber toe—and went for a run. When I got back to our apartment at the university I did what I still believe was the key to my having stuck with it now all these years. Without showering, without changing, I sat down at the typewriter and started typing—whatever came to mind, whatever I could remember of the run. I didn't do it on purpose, I just did it. But it quickly became habit, and I did it again and again for fifteen, sixteen months. It was some combination of running and typing, of remembering Dad on that walk and myself on that hill that unlocked the secret of making "road work" somehow doable.

These first Alaska runs had little rhyme or reason. They were just runs, out the door. The university maintains a well-groomed network of cross-country ski trails, and during the summer they offered miles of opportunities through the birch and pine trees. Every so often I added to the distance. There was no set pattern, no grand plan, except that when I got back home I typed. It was months before I replaced the sneakers with actual running shoes. Eventually I wanted a goal, a larger reason, something less about Dad and the past and more about me and the present. If you live in Fairbanks, Alaska, and you desire purpose on the run, there is only one choice: the Equinox Marathon.

I have watched New England's Joan Benoit win the Boston Marathon; stood in the shadow of the Los Angeles Coliseum when Portugal's thirty-seven-year-old Carlos Lopes ran away with the 1984 Olympic gold medal; walked to Fourth Avenue in Brooklyn time and again for the New York Marathon, the city's best day of the year. Nothing compares with the Equinox Marathon in Fairbanks, Alaska.

The race started in 1963, more of a hike than an actual competition. Nat Goodhue, one of the course designers, won the men's division that first year in 3 hours, 52 minutes, and 22 seconds. Another designer, Gail Bakken, won the women's race in 6 hours, 8 minutes. The clockings only seem unimpressive. The Equinox was expressly designed to challenge not time but terrain. Utilizing many of the ski trails, the course climbs from barely 600 feet at mile eight up the side of Ester Dome to nearly 2,400 feet by about the twelve-and-half-mile mark. From there it's three miles down and back up the far side of the dome, through a trio of up-and-down treks before diving off the face of the earth (it seems) straight down the quarter-mile Alder Chute at the beginning of a five-mile quad-crushing downhill to mile twenty-two, back at 600 feet. Get that far and it's only four more flattish miles. It is an awful race; it is a fabulous race. Fairbanksans for whom the Equinox is their *raison de running* are rightfully proud of the course and the accomplishment that awaits them—and they are fiercely protective of both. If you run in Alaska's interior, the Equinox calls your name.

I had another reason to climb Ester Dome and throw myself off. The friend with me on the pipeline hike, Bob Murphy, was already a two-time Equinox winner. Murph's father died of a heart attack in 1960. He was fifty years old. Murph was seven; his older brother, Billy, nine; their younger sister, Ann, five. The family was fishing off the Capitola Pier, a couple of miles from their cottage in Santa Cruz, California, when Mr. Murphy said they needed to get home. More alarming, he asked his wife, Ann, to drive. Mr. Murphy always drove. Back at the cottage he said he needed to lie down. The kids "got shepherded out of the house, down to a neighbor," Murph remembers. At some point a priest showed up and an ambulance was called. "The next thing we knew, there's Dad getting carried out of the house."

Murph and Billy started running in the mid-1970s. Murph says his Dad's fate was clearly a factor in his getting going. "It's always in the back of my mind," he says, though the running success he has since come to enjoy has become its own reward, freeing him from the memory. As for Billy: "Dad has always been part of the equation." In any event, running looked like fun, and, as it turned out, Billy and Bobby Murphy were both pretty good at it. In 1977, Billy ran "The Ave"—the Avenue of the Giants Marathon—through Humboldt Redwoods State Park in California, finishing in 2 hours, 51 minutes, less than half an hour behind the winner. That same year Murph ran his first Equinox. He led to the top of the Dome but was unsure how far down the back he had to run. A rookie mistake and it cost him; he faded badly and finished tenth.

Murph and his girlfriend, Claire Rudolf, from Spokane, Washington, had been Jesuit Volunteers out at St. Mary's with Noreen and me. They moved to Fairbanks in 1977, and it was in large measure because of them that Noreen and I followed in August 1978. That September, Murph ran his second Equinox. He made no mistakes.

The course record was 2:53:59, set by Olé Kristiansen in 1976. Olé had been the university's ski coach, and the old-timers talked of him in reverent tones. His time had sheared nearly six minutes off the previous record, and he had won by more than thirteen. The consensus held that his mark was untouchable, likely forever. When Murph set off on a sub-2:50 pace, the disbelief was palpable, a barely concealed chuckle. There was no way this guy in yellow shorts and white singlet with the black "Rocky" T-shirt underneath could keep this up.

The climb would get him. The dome would get him. The turn-around would get him. The run down would get him. *Something* would get him. But nothing did.

I have attended three Olympics, an NCAA Final Four, the Super Bowl, any number of big-time games. No event will ever match that 1978 small-town Equinox in pure excitement and for my complete, visceral attachment to it. Never have I wished more passionately for an outcome. Murph was perfectly suited to the running game, a joy to watch. At 5-foot-8, maybe 125 pounds, what there was of him was all lungs and legs and heart, his feet nearly smacking him in the butt as his strides ate up the ground. He was a voracious hill climber, an Equinox prerequisite, but just as important he was durable on the downhill, which can turn quadriceps into concrete. Win or lose he was gracious and good natured, an old-fashioned sportsman, but underneath he was fiercely competitive and totally dedicated.

Midway through the race, before Murph had even reached the top of Ester Dome, it was obvious this was his to win. At least it was to us, his camp followers—Claire, Noreen and me, Jim and Chris Villano, another husband and wife originally from St. Mary's, and the Jesuit Volunteer Corps. Billy was there as well. With his girlfriend, Mary, they had hitchhiked up from San Francisco. Keeping up with a marathoner—driving ahead to the next checkpoint; fretting that you'll miss him—is great, frenetic fun. That we were following the leader just whipped it to a froth.

Billy and his gorgeous, high-strung Irish setter, Sara, went solo in Murph's blue Volkswagen van. The rest of us trailed as best we could. Billy had warned us the night before, sort of joking, to stay out of his way during the race. Billy and Bobby were preternaturally close. You could tell they shared an exceptional bond, forged perhaps by that common experience of years ago. In the days before the race the brothers had run various sections of the course together, plotting strategy, and now their moment had arrived. When the starting gun sounded, Billy took off for the blue van, Sara bounding next to him, his own race to the first checkpoint already on. Billy was coach, strategist, water boy, *domestique*. When the old-timers guarding the status quo were out of earshot (and sometimes when they weren't) he was his brother's staunchest defender as well, spouting profane, they-can-stick-their-record adjurations. His infectious, unabashed energy fueled the day, sparked the excitement, raised the stakes. Billy Murphy made the Equinox Marathon matter.

Well before the finish, the only remaining questions were by how much Murph would lower the current mark and how soundly he would beat the second-place runner. With about eight miles left we caught up to him on Henderson Road. I remember the particulars. The gray, overcast sky. The pine trees an almost black-green as winter approached, a scant few gold leaves still clinging to the birches. And then the Brothers Murphy came pounding down the road, a hard-packed dirt back then, stride for stride, their footfalls slapping the air. They ran past us, Billy handing Murph a water bottle, spewing encouragement and split times and pieces of strategy. Murph was going to win! It remains as thrilling a sports moment as I have ever witnessed.

We got to the finish a few minutes before Murph. He would break free of the trees at the far end of the athletic field for the final 200 yards. One of the old guard sauntered over to Billy and asked—meekly, apologetically—what kind of time to expect from his brother. But Billy was having none of this change of heart, this coming over to the bright side. "He's going to crush it," he yelled, in one final uncontainable burst. "He's going to crush it!" With that Murph popped from the trees and into the clearing. He won in 2:48:20, shattering the record by five minutes, thirty-nine seconds, virtually matching Olé's dominance. And he won by more than seven minutes, in the process pulling both the second- and third-place finishers under the magic three-hour barrier for the first time.

For all that, it would take years for me to fully appreciate that 1978 race, to find the words to explain its significance. Actually, I never did. I must borrow from Jim Villano. That Equinox was on the third Saturday in September. Noreen and I had been married barely two months. While not new to Alaska, we were to Fairbanks, a middle-of-nowhere outpost where in winter the mercury would drop to 45- or 50-below zero. Noreen had found a job at the university; I was hoping that a temporary gig as jack of all trades with a local bush airline might turn permanent. We were living at John Ringstadt's house, a friend of a friend, who had offered us his place when a job had suddenly materialized for him out in Kotzebue, north of the Arctic Circle. Our world was unknown and brand new, wildly exciting, totally unnerving. For Jim and Chris and their baby, Lisa, it was much the same. Years later, remembering Murph's first Equinox win, Jim told me how that victory had filled him with a confidence he maybe didn't know he had. That if Murph could triumph, maybe Jim could, too, as he started out on this new life thousands of miles from Fort Lee, New Jersey, where he'd grown up. Yes, that says it.

For me to get to my own Equinox triumph, or at least some personal victory, I first had to run through one of those Fairbanks winters. This was both easier said than done and not hard at all. Turned out I loved running in the Fairbanks cold. I relished the challenge and looked forward to the ritual of getting dressed to get out. Ever since there has been no end-of-workout satisfaction quite to match the moment when the run was done at 35 below, my layers of clothes were a sodden mess, and I had to gingerly peel the stocking cap off my face because it had frozen into my beard.

Large-mesh fishnet underwear went on first, to create a layer of air between the skin and the regular lightweight long underwear that went on next. Thin knee-high wool socks over that. Sweat pants. Turtleneck sweater. Lightweight vest (a cutoff sweatshirt sufficed). Over it all a creamsicle-colored thigh-length cloth (for breathability) rain jacket a size too big, even on me. A thin stocking cap with face mask pulled over my head and tucked into my turtleneck; a thicker wool cap pulled down over my ears. A pair of mittens (light as possible; my hands rarely got cold). Around my face a scarf that smelled of damp sheep and yesterday's sweat, my intimate companions on today's run. Finally, over it all, a large plastic-mesh Alaska Department of Transportation orange-and-yellow reflective vest. By the time I was done with the run, the vest would be frozen stiff around me, my armor against the night.

Now it was out the door quickly. This was the beauty of it; once suited, you couldn't dally, you had to get out there and get going before a layer of sweat chilled you. Despite all of that there was still a shock of the cold when you hit it. A good thing, this. Your body was soon to be a raging furnace. When you stopped, you could see the steam rising off yourself. So if at first you didn't feel the cold, you were overdressed. Really.

Fairbanks sits in a valley. During the winter, temperature inversions—warm air above trapping cold air below—camp over the city. Ice fog, the disingenuous name for the smog of frozen carbon monoxide from car exhaust, envelops the place. I see the time and temperature blinking on the bank clock at the corner of College Avenue and Farmer's Loop Road, just off the hill from the university: "3:45 P.M." (and pitch black); "-42°" (in the Alaskan interior, fortunately, there is rarely wind chill). That's the coldest I remember running in. And I admit I did it so I could say I did it. But 30-, 35-below zero was a regular day, sometimes for days on end. If I wasn't willing, I would go weeks without running at all.

I never felt the risk of the cold was unreasonable. Of more concern, I always believed, was the darkness, which was why the reflective vest. That and I couldn't wear my glasses—they immediately frosted over—making my runs an indiscernible blur. As for all those clothes, you got used to it, however difficult that is to believe in an era of moisture-wicking threads and ultralight synthetics. Anyway, you didn't so much wear the clothes as the clothes wore you. Like with the oversized clown suit on the actor Bill Irwin, they were only along for the ride, flopping and flouncing as you ran around inside them.

Best of it all about running in the super cold was the sound. There was first the *frumph-frumph-frumphing* of all that fabric once you found the rhythm of your run. And the cold itself created its own consonance. Robert Service wrote of it as "a silence you most could *hear.*" That's the poet's italics. Running on packed snow in sub-zero temperatures is to run across a giant (and cheap) Styrofoam cooler. The colder the air the shriller the squeal of your shoes on its surface, and the more hollow it feels. No way it should support, yet it does.

That was just the half of it. A temperature inversion confines more than just the cold beneath the warm. It also traps sound. This warmer "roof" prevents it from dissipating. With the thermal layer sometimes only twenty feet off the ground, noise takes on an astounding resonance. Running on a road outside Fairbanks at 35-below, I could hear a car distinctly even when its lights were still just a glow on the horizon. As it approached, I could differentiate the engine's RPMs from the tires' grip on the road. Once the car was upon me, the noise was a single mass, screaming at me, ear-splitting and teeth-rattling, as loud as a jet engine.

I didn't remember that I hadn't forgotten this until Tuesday, September 11, 2001, at 9:03 A.M.—nineteen years since my last Fairbanks winter. I was at the corner of South End Avenue and Albany Street in New York City, two blocks south and one block west of the World Trade Center, running away from an inflamed North Tower and the *Wall Street Journal* offices across Liberty Street from it. I couldn't see the second plane, but I could hear it, a terrible shriek overwhelming the tip of

Manhattan, obliterating all other life. This was no Golden Oldie on a baby boomer radio station, but it was soundtrack nonetheless. In the final few seconds before the deep-throated impact returned to me the present, I was back in Fairbanks, out in the cold, lost in a run.

━━━━━

I should listen to Kathy and let go of Dad and his cigarettes, if only because he never could. But the two are so inextricably bound. For all I know, he left one burning in the ashtray by the sofa on that Tuesday night in 1969.

After Dad's heart attack in 1963, if there was any hope to be had at all, any silver lining in this dark cough of a cloud that had crashed upon us, it was that now for sure Dad would give up smoking. He had to know he had to quit, didn't he? But he never did. Oh, he stopped for a while, but that's all it ever was. A temporary ceasefire, like we were hearing about constantly from Vietnam. You always knew it would flare up again. Dad never stopped thinking like a smoker, even if I don't know what a smoker thinks like. The heart attack was in February. By the summer he was back at work, which meant he was back to the cigarettes. A equaled B. Getting Dad "back on his feet," back to work, was surely the right thing to do. If I can't picture Dad without a cigarette, it is equally impossible to imagine him without Cole Steel. He needed his job, he was his job. That was the correct therapy, getting him back to work. But it was also the only therapy we had. And at his job he smoked.

It was Dad's doctor who gave him the go-ahead, Mom says. Dad was back at Cole Steel full time, walking the warehouse, talking to New York, keeping forklifts in tire treads. At one of his regular checkups with the doctor, Dad said that a cigarette would, you know, sure feel good once in a while. And the doctor said, well, you know, if you think a smoke now and again might take the edge off, what's the harm? That's all Dad needed. *The doctor said I could.*

Mom says she always assumed the doctor couldn't have been a smoker himself. Only a nonsmoker would tell a smoker that "once in a while" wouldn't hurt. A smoker would know better. But many years later, Mom says, she was on a bus outing with a group of fellow seniors. The doctor was in the front row, and at the first stop he bolted with a few others, reaching with the rest of them for the cigarette pack. Maybe he wasn't a smoker in 1969. Or maybe he was worried about losing Dad's business. He had been Dad's doc since I can't remember. He was a good man, he deserves his due, fully dedicated, the old-fashioned country doctor who made house calls. But surely he knew his patient. If he had told Dad to quit—*give 'em up, Red, they're gonna kill ya*—Dad would have walked. The doctor knew what I refuse to know, even now. Dad had to smoke. (If the doctor did smoke, the cigarettes never really got him; he died in 2004, at age eighty.)

It was lung cancer—not heart disease—that raised the flags back then, the warning signs hoisted since the nineteenth century was rolling into the twentieth. There are references to cigarettes as "coffin nails" as far back as the 1890s. Statistically, lung cancer didn't really exist until cigarettes provided the cheap, convenient, and efficient (not to mention wildly popular) delivery system for tobacco's smoke. But it wasn't until the late

1940s—when 44 percent of all Americans eighteen years of age or older smoked, according to a Gallup poll—that the idea that cigarettes might not be a good thing gained any traction. Independently, three studies in 1950 correlated smoking to lung cancer, the preponderance of evidence finally moving the needle. One of the studies, in fact, used data collected from patients at what was then Roswell Park Memorial Institute, in Buffalo. The statistics reached back at least a decade, to a day when Dad's Western New York body might still have been smoke free.

That lung cancer (and not heart disease) was the leading concern makes sense. Until Dad's first coronary, I'm sure that was our family's thinking as well. Smoke gets in your lungs. The realization that the heart was at risk was as inevitable as an iceberg, but the reasoning was also about as fast moving. This is particularly frustrating now, because in hindsight it all seems so obvious. In fact, it was the American Cancer Society, in a 1954 preliminary report of a large study on death rates and smoking habits, that sounded a first warning about smoking and the heart. Then in September 1955, President Dwight Eisenhower suffered a myocardial infarction while in Denver. Eisenhower had been a four-pack-a-day Camel man, though he had quit cold turkey in 1949, the general appalled at the lack of discipline the "cancer sticks" exposed. Dad liked Ike; he voted for him twice. In 1956, the American Heart Association weighed in with an opinion, though it basically just called for more study; a 1960 report would contain more bite. In 1961, the now-famous Framingham Heart Study introduced what it called "factors of risk" into the national vocabulary (blood pressure and cholesterol). *Reader's Digest* had for years been holding the tobacco industry's feet to the fire; an article in November 1962 titled "DANGER: *Smoke at Your Own Risk!*" said in the introduction that "more cigarette smokers die of heart disease associated with smoking than die of lung cancer." And of course in 1964 the advisory committee to the Surgeon General released its landmark report on smoking and health. Twelve paragraphs addressed the coronary question. Not until 1968 (in a supplement to a 1967 report) would the heart issue be directly tackled. By the mid-1960s Congress would act to put warning labels on cigarette packs; by the end of the decade, the tobacco industry, bowing to the inevitable, would voluntarily agree to stop advertising on TV. Through it all, Dad smoked. And I was desperate for him to stop. Through it all, cardiovascular disease remained America's number one killer. It would be facile of me to say now that I knew then that cigarettes would get him. But I did. Why didn't he?

At the McKee household in York, Pennsylvania, in the 1950s and 1960s, the news arrived via four sources. There was the *York Dispatch*, the local evening paper. There was NBC's evening news on WGAL-TV Channel 8 in Lancaster. Our first TV was this huge, black thing that hulked in the corner. Dad once tried to move it and ended up in York Hospital for a hernia operation. Kathy and I were too young to get in then, so Mom drove us to the parking lot and we got out and waved to him at the window, ten, twelve stories up. *The Huntley-Brinkley Report* was on through the 1960s, but in 1956 (our first television year) there was still the *Camel News Caravan* (sponsored by the cigarette) with John Cameron

Swayze, soon to become the Cole Steel typewriter spokesman and, more famously, Timex watch pitchman. There was also *LIFE* magazine. Mom's Early American tinker's bench coffee table was never without a few issues. But mostly there was *TIME* magazine. *TIME* was everywhere. In the bathroom, next to the sofa, stacked in the basement.

I see Dad reading *TIME*, and I wonder what early-warning articles he might have read and chosen to ignore. The Internet renders that speculation easily enough satisfied.

A short piece early on said that the *Journal of the American Medical Association*'s "one hard & fast conclusion is that doctors should do much more research into the effect of smoking on the heart and arteries." That was in the November 17, 1952, *TIME*—the day I was born. Eisenhower's heart attack in 1955 presaged an avalanche of coverage, including a *TIME* cover story on Halloween. "[H]eart disease is still medicine's most stubborn mystery," it surmised, correctly.

Another cover story, on January 13, 1961, talked inside about "That Remarkable Cholesterol," a word soon to be heard regularly at our house, after Dad's first attack. And in an article on September 1, 1967, reporting on a Senate subcommittee hearing on the progress toward an effective cigarette filter, the eighth paragraph began, "Nicotine demonstrably places dangerous strain upon the heart muscles."

There are more where those came from, of course. (The *Reader's Digest* article mentioned above, for instance, was condensed from the July 6, 1962, *TIME*.) But citing them here would assuage only me. Besides, legitimate science and the cigarette monolith had only just begun in earnest their dance of death; there were many years to go before the denouement to come. It does leave one to wonder, though, what obvious conclusions we should be gleaning from today's various debates, rather than waiting forty-plus years to lament why we didn't act sooner.

The years I researched also include the moment of the great transplant breakthroughs. A fact I had forgotten, though I shouldn't have: on December 15, 1967, Dr. Christiaan Barnard received cover acclaim for the first-ever successful heart transplant. One year later, *TIME* would declare that in the past dozen months "95 human hearts have been taken from newly dead donors and implanted in the chests of 93 patients (two of them got two apiece)."

I should have remembered that era, because I have to wonder if Dad hadn't already signed on with it. To that moment when the great promise of science had blown past the more pedestrian ideas of prevention, never to be headed again. Dad was a big believer in education, its potential and possibilities. For instance, he delighted in my abilities with "Plastic Bricks," and how I could build multistory skyscrapers, each of the three or four levels more compact than the one below it. *Engineering!* he always declared when I had completed another, *the future is in engineering!* Perhaps he felt that way about his heart. That science would find a way. Hadn't it once already, with the atom bomb? Indeed, in a *TIME* essay in the February 25, 1966, issue titled "The Futurists: Looking Toward A.D. 2000" the McKee magazine of record declared that "[p]robably arteriosclerotic heart disease will also have been eliminated" by the turn of the coming century.

TIME suggests one other explanation for Dad's attitude. The Surgeon General's advisory committee released its cautiously worded 1964 report on smoking and health on January 11, a Saturday, so as not to roil the financial markets. *TIME*, likely working against a deadline, devoted less than a full page to the story in its January 17 issue. (*LIFE*, on the other hand, covered it exhaustively across eleven: "Verdict on Cigarets: Guilty as Charged.") The next week *TIME* came back with coverage of the press coverage. It included a selection of the political cartoons of the moment. One, by Gene Basset of the *New York World-Telegram,* shows a man, his arms folded, one hand ponderously on his chin, contemplating the pack of cigarettes on the table before him. I can conjure Dad in that man: the hair, the suit, the white shirt, the too-large nose. The caption reads: "MOMENT OF TRUTH *Seven out of ten gave up reading.*"

The only props I will allow Dad is that at least he smoked back in a day when everybody did. Virtually all of my parents' friends smoked. I spent my childhood enveloped in second-hand smoke. I would say everything and everybody smelled of smoke, except back then who could have noticed? Among the members of Mom and Dad's most immediate circle of perhaps twelve, fourteen St. Joe's couples, I can say with certainty that only two people didn't smoke. Ashtrays were a necessary decorative element in every house. I have spoken with the survivors about those old days. To a person, there was a helpless shrug of the shoulder when I asked why they smoked, followed by a meek, "Everybody did." Though as one York dad pointed out,

I was asking the wrong question. Smoking is addictive, he said. That's *why* they smoked. "The real question is, 'Why did we start?'" And with that he meekly shrugged his shoulders. "Because everybody did."

Everybody doesn't smoke now; but too many people still do. In the summer of 1969, 40 percent of Americans eighteen and older smoked. Today that number is down to 21 percent. That's still more than one in five. And the decline itself is deceiving, because in the past few years it has been leveling off. Meanwhile, if the bar is lowered to include everyone twelve years of age and up, the number jumps to nearly one in four. More than four of ten adults age eighteen to twenty-five use a tobacco product. Among kids twelve to seventeen, the statistics are encouraging in one light: "only" 10.8 percent of these kids smoke, and the rate is declining. On the other hand, among high-school age kids, that number is 23 percent. Every day about 3,900 kids twelve to seventeen give smoking a shot; for 1,500 it becomes a daily thing. Native Americans, meanwhile, have far and away the highest smoking rates in the country, at nearly 40 percent; having lived in rural Alaska, I can attest to that. And cigarettes are horrifically insidious: The less educated a person is, the more likely he or she is to smoke. A person without a job is more likely to be a smoker than is a person with one. Smoking costs this country $92 billion annually in lost productivity and $75.5 billion in healthcare. Approximately one-third of people who smoke can expect their death to be directly related to it. Cigarettes remain the number one cause of preventable death. Find distance from that sentence and its reality shivers. *Preventable death*. That means they didn't have to die. Not now, not like this. On average, smokers die thirteen to fourteen years earlier than nonsmokers. They could have lived longer; met their grandkids; grown old with a spouse.

Once on a St. Patrick's Day, Mom and Dad had many of their St. Joe's friends over to the house ahead of the parish dance. They were great entertainers, Helen and Red. There were the usual drinks, the usual cigarettes, a few cigars. Lots of laughs. As with every party, the living room slowly blurred beneath a grayish haze, thicker with every lighted match. One of Dad's regular hosting duties was to make periodic circles with the silent butler emptying the ashtrays. It was snowing, and as they were preparing to leave, a call came in that the dance had been postponed, so everyone settled back for another round and more smokes. Still, the party broke up early enough that Kathy and I weren't in bed when everyone left. It was then that we noticed that our bird, a beautiful orange-yellow canary that liked to sing to the whistling tea kettle, appeared not to be in its cage, hung near the ceiling between the living and dining rooms. Dad got up on a chair, and we watched him reach into the cage and pull out a limp handful of feathers. Dad ran for the kitchen door, to fresh air, grabbing a bottle of whiskey on the way. Kathy and I stood in the hallway, horrified, as Dad bobbed its beak with a bit of booze, snow swirling in the back porch light. The bird let out a terrible shriek that sent Kathy and me running down the hall. Then there was silence, no sound at all. The canary in our coal mine, dead.

WEDNESDAY,
OCTOBER 1; 9:00 A.M.

No way I wanted to see this. By the time I ran out of the house last night after the ambulance showed up, to get to Mom down at Schmitts, the TV room was well trashed. The blanket on the green carpet smeared with some of the foamy stuff from Dad's mouth, two of the sofa cushions thrown aside, Dad slumped on the third in a dark stain of his own wetness. I did not want to go back in there.

Mom and I had spent the night up at Philbins, their house at the top of Haines Acres with the picture window looking over all of York. Once we left the hospital we had gone back to Schmitts; Mom had been there playing bridge with Mrs. Schmitt, Mrs. Malloy, and Mrs. Anderson. But not long after, once a couple of the other St. Joe's moms had come over for awhile, Mom said she wanted to go up to Philbins for the night.

Within the York Crowd there were various pairings, and McKee-Philbin is one. Few of the York Crowd houses were ever locked. And while at some you had to knock first and wait for the door to open, or knock while you opened the door yourself, with the Philbins and McKees, you just pushed the door open and walked in, declaring your presence as you did. Other families probably had this same kind of arrangement with other families. Everyone knew—just knew.

Dad taught Mr. Philbin to fly-fish. They'd sometimes take off on a Sunday afternoon, too late to get their lines wet, but with enough daylight to go look at the water. Just look at the water. The two of them once even finagled this on Mother's Day, getting both families piled into two cars to go take a gander at the Susquehanna River. "That was a good trick," Mr. Philbin says with a laugh.

Mom and Mrs. Philbin spent many, many hours together. Sometimes with Mrs. Flick they went into business together, one time making and selling Heritage Wreaths out of pine cones that we kids would gather out at Sam Lewis State Park. Mrs. Philbin was from a large Philadelphia Irish Catholic family—irreverent, brassy ("earthy," as she preferred it), easy to laugh, "Jesus, Mary, and Joseph!" her all-purpose phrase. She had carte blanche to give me a stern word or a quick back of her hand if she thought I needed it. Like with the door-opening agreements, Mom and Mrs. Philbin likely never discussed this, at least not in so many words; it just grew with the friendship over the years.

And now that friendship had come to this. Mom and me and Mrs. Philbin and her older daughter, Gail, a senior with me at York Catholic, sitting in the Philbins' kitchen after midnight in a hushed and darkened house. Pat and Dennis and Mary Eileen and Jeff were asleep upstairs, Jimmy away at school. Mr. Philbin wasn't home; he was on a business trip. I wished he were here; I wanted him here. Dad was gone; not

Mr. Philbin, too. At Schmitts, Mrs. Masterson had said that Mr. Masterson was away on business, out in Chicago. That was three dads not here, and I could feel the absence, every one. For reasons I can't explain, this remains my most vivid sensation of that night, once I ran from our house. Too many fathers missing. Gail must have felt it, too. "I wish Dad was here," she said, cutting the kitchen quiet.

Now it was morning. Mom had pulled the Cutlass into the driveway, and it was time to go back into our house. I let her go first, by a couple of minutes. There was just no way. Eventually though, I knew I had to get out of the car, walk across the slab of front-porch concrete with the crack across the middle, and open the door and walk in. When I did, there was Mom, still framed in the doorway between foyer and TV room, staring in the direction of the sofa. I froze for a moment but then walked up behind her and looked in.

The place was immaculate, clean from top to bottom, sofa put together, urine stain disappeared, blanket gone, ashtrays emptied. On closer inspection—I looked, wandering around the house—it was obvious the vacuum had been run. Not just in the TV room but the living and dining rooms as well. I could see the tracks. In the kitchen, any stray dishes Mom hadn't gotten to last night were washed, dried, and put away. Then I looked in the refrigerator. It was packed, totally stocked. Milk, eggs, cheese, butter; ice cream in the freezer. That prompted me to open the cupboards. Filled.

We never learned who did this. Was it a single person, one thoughtful mom? A mom and dad on their own? Perhaps a couple of people had shown up unplanned and unannounced.

The door was unlocked, that's for sure. Or maybe once the news got out—and I had seen how quickly that could travel—a battle plan was implemented. I'll get this; you do that; we're on our way to the store. Mom never found out and she never asked. She already knew the answer: the York Crowd.

———

They came from everywhere, these York Crowd people, from as close as Steelton, near Harrisburg; and Lancaster, across the Susquehanna River; and as far away as Chicago; St. Louis; The Bronx; Philadelphia; Wheeler, West Virginia; Dayton; Worcester, Massachusetts; Los Angeles; Pittsburgh; Peoria; and Buffalo. They came from everywhere to York, and not just York but to East York, not just East York but to Springettsbury Township, and not just Springettsbury Township but to St. Joseph's parish, the most important destination of all.

York has always been a crossroads town, connecting north to south. The Monocacy Indian Path forded the Codorus Creek in what is now downtown, on the way to the Cumberland Gap. A map from the 1770s shows seven roads in and out. Market Street itself is Old Lincoln Highway. The city's finest hour might have come in the winter of 1777-78. With General Washington encamped at Valley Forge, the Continental Congress meanwhile had retreated west across the Susquehanna to "York Town" to escape the British in Philadelphia. While in the White Rose City the Congress adopted the Articles of Confederation. I always include "first capital of the United States" when bragging on York to people who have never heard of the place, though it's more marketing slogan than truth.

The city's relationship to the Civil War is murkier. York, only fifteen miles from Maryland, behaved very much like a Border State during the War of Northern Aggression: part of the Union; not unsympathetic to the Confederacy. The whole unpleasantness was someone else's problem—the most-unpopular Lincoln's—until the conflict came to York. In the final days of June 1863, with the opposing armies being pulled inexorably to the great conflagration at Gettysburg, the Confederate infantry of Maj. Gen. Jubal A. Early neared York. City fathers hastily assembled a delegation that rode out to intercept and parley a deal. Exact intentions remain in debate. A wise recognition of the inevitable? Or a too-eager concession? Later, when Confederate Brig. Gen. John Brown Gordon was riding through town, a young girl handed him flowers—with a concealed note detailing the whereabouts of the Union troops at Wrightsville and the strategic Susquehanna River bridge. It was at the time the largest covered span in the world, and retreating Union troops were forced to torch it to prevent Early from continuing on to Harrisburg. The gala pageant at the fairgrounds in 1966 celebrating York's 225th anniversary included the flower-girl encounter. I remember because I was appalled to learn it.

The English and the Scots-Irish helped settle York County, but it was the oppressed peoples of the Palatinate along the Rhine in Germany and Switzerland who put their stamp on the region, coming in large numbers to southeast Pennsylvania, originally at the urging of William Penn. Adjectives like "solid," "hardworking," and "industrious" are frequently used to describe them.

York County is carpeted in rich agricultural land, but the city itself has long existed to make things. Codorus Furnace out near the Susquehanna River resupplied the Continental Army after the Valley Forge winter. It was owned for a time by York's James Smith, a signer of the Declaration of Independence. The first iron steamboat in the United States was built in York; so was the first coal-fired steam locomotive, a few years later in 1831. For about fifteen years in the early days of the twentieth century, the Pullman Motor Car Company of York produced luxury automobiles, beginning with an innovative (if ultimately impractical) six-wheeler. For a time there were even two car makers in town. By December 7, 1941, York boasted a broad industrial base, and World War II ensured that the city would be a driving engine of the postwar boom. Anchored by companies like York Ice Machinery Corporation, area manufacturers devised a cooperative strategy to keep all the factories humming on defense contracts. "The York Plan," as it came to be called, would be copied during the war by communities across the country. As a result, by the late 1940s and early 1950s a well-located York could brag of a highly skilled, experienced workforce. Just as important, there was room to grow—for factories, shopping centers, housing tracts.

Grow it did. In the dozen or so years from the early 1950s to the mid-1960s, the York Crowd dads moved in to work at Top Flite Tape, York Narrow Fabrics, Bendix, Standard Register, Noonan Construction, Shiny Brite, Maple Press, Lyon Metals, Glidden, General Tire, GTE Sylvania, Cole Steel, and Caterpillar. Many of these companies were long established; others were, like all of the dads, new to York. The boom was on. There were about 200,000 people in York County in 1950. By 1960 there would be an additional 36,000; by 1970, 34,000 more; by 1980, 40,000 on top of that.

If Helen O'Neil and John McKee were part of the Buffalo exodus, they were very nearly charter members in York's postwar expansion. We McKees arrived in February 1954. We came, of course, because of Cole Steel, always Cole Steel. But Dad also wanted out of New York City. Mom and Dad had been living on Second Avenue downtown when Kathy was born in 1949. When I came along in 1952 they were in Paramus, New Jersey, in a tiny house of their own, Dad a soldier in the commuter army.

John J. McKee, junior executive, was thrilled to be in York. He had to be. He wasn't in New York. He had a great job at a great company with a great future, arriving only a few years after the company itself had come to town. And there was terrific hunting and fishing everywhere around him—within walking distance, it must have seemed. For Mom it was different. They first rented a house on a peacock farm out in Dover, northwest of York (fifty years later the question of Intelligent Design being mentioned in the public schools would come to trial there). With Dad eagerly off to his career each day, Mom, with no car, sat on a farm with a four-year-old girl and a fifteen-month-old baby boy, the nearest house maybe a mile away. Mom still speaks of an early-spring day, the weather having finally broke, when she gussied herself up and paraded off to the neighbor lady with an apple pie offering, Kathy by the hand, me in the pram. The screen door remained shut. A few words through the wire mesh, and that was that. Mom left, devastated.

If York was a small town in the 1950s, it was not uncomplicated. If only because no place is. The 1950 city directory inadvertently explains the why of it: "Without any influx of a trouble-making European element, York has remained truly American in ideals and habits of living." Well, those days were over. York was soon to be teeming with people who weren't . . . Yorkers. The city was being pushed and pulled, molded and shaped (bent, folded, and mutilated, some surely thought) by an outside world that had moved in and wasn't leaving.

Nothing defines this dynamic more dramatically than Caterpillar. The heavy-equipment company from Peoria, Illinois, came to East York in 1952, buying up 200 acres of an old hog farm north of East Market Street, and opening for business late the next year. Its monstrous compound would eventually enclose about 1.5 million square feet of round-the-clock manufacturing. By the late 1960s, CAT in York was providing for all of Caterpillar's service centers west to Pittsburgh, north into Canada, south to Florida, plus South America and Western Europe. It employed nearly 4,000 people, paid good money, provided great benefits, and offered generous vacations. CAT also helped do precisely what the naysayers said it would: it inflated York's wage scale, drained existing industries of their best workers, and flooded York County with thousands of new families. When Caterpillar finally shut down most of its York operations in the late 1990s after a final few years of struggle, not everyone considered it a sad day.

Mom says that when she and Dad were looking to buy a house in 1954, Realtors were funneling all up-and-coming middle-class customers to East York. For that reason only did we move clear across York County to Wilshire Drive, out east. A three-bedroom, one-bath ranch with an unfinished basement dying to be fixed up plus a huge backyard bordered by rows of thick, lush snowball spirea that exploded white every May. Dad used it to make a floral crown when it was my turn to crown the Blessed Mother in first grade. Mom and Dad signed the papers on their $16,900 dream on Monday, November 8, their seventh wedding anniversary. That not a month after Willie Mays of the New York Giants had run down an impossibly long fly ball in the center-field canyon at the Polo Grounds in Game One of the World Series with his famous over-the-shoulder catch. The ball was hit by Vic Wertz, a Cleveland Indian, born in York, another bit of local braggadocio.

That we were now in St. Joseph's parish was pure accident. Or maybe not. York was not a Catholic town. In 1950 there were sixty-seven churches in York, four of them Catholic; there were eighteen religious denominations, one of them Catholic. The math on either is less than 6 percent. Some would say York was anti-Catholic. I have listened to old-time Yorkers tell stories of being kids and sitting on a hill south of York watching the Ku Klux Klan burn crosses on the hillside across the valley. A York Crowd dad says that before he moved to York a work colleague who had already made the jump got an urgent, two-word message to him: "Don't come." The dad came anyway.

They all did. It's where the jobs were. But if York was not a Catholic town, growing up I never knew it.

By the time we got to St. Joseph Church on Princess Street, the parish was already on its second house of worship, dedicated in May 1954. The first was built in 1909 in what was then called "Bull Frog Alley," an area settled by Gypsy families in the 1800s. The 1954 structure was the first church building in York of completely modern design, its roof and steeple all angles and edges and flat-planed surfaces. Inside, a huge oak arch dominated the wall behind the altar, soaring to the ceiling. Nestled within it was a life-size, wood-carved figure of Christ on a mahogany cross. In school, one of the St. Francis sisters advised us to think of the arch as a pair of folded hands praying to God. Another said the arch was a boat, and we were all with Jesus sailing off to heaven.

Amen. My First Communion and Confirmation; every year the Holy Thursday and Good Friday services; the Stations of the Cross Friday afternoons during Lent; the May procession; Forty Hours, with its Litany of the Saints raced through at breakneck speed in Latin by fifty, sixty diocesan priests (the response *Ora pro nobis* sounded like "ol' rotten oranges"). During school air-raid practice we would all scurry across the parking lot and into the church, where we'd sit scrunched into the pews as far from the center aisle as we could get, reciting the rosary. When the bombs came, we'd be saved because the ceiling would collapse into the middle, sparing us pressed to the walls . . . which would remain standing. St. Joe's would save us. And like Dad, because of Dad, I was an altar boy until my junior year in high school. I enjoyed it thoroughly and quit

only because a priest who was all of maybe 5-foot-4 transferred in and next to him my 6-feet-8-inches and 160 pounds
felt suddenly freakish and ridiculous. When Noreen and I
were married there in 1978, our best man, Joe McMenamin, a
friend since York Catholic, was forty-five minutes late flying up
from Atlanta, where he was doing his residency. I marked time
in the sacristy, the mixed aroma of charcoal, incense, and
heavy-coated waxed candles familiar and calming.

Sunday at St. Joe's meant seeing the York Crowd. It's why I
went to church—I mean, besides the fact that I had to go,
there was no question I would go, it was a mortal sin if I didn't
go. All of the families would be there. Not just there but almost in assigned seats. The Flicks and their six kids. The Mastersons and their six (one still to come). The Schmitts and their
six over here; the Philbins and their six over there. The McEntees and their five. On and on, they were everywhere. Later, in
college, home for a weekend, when I could probably have not
gone to church had I told Mom so, I still went . . . because I
knew I'd see everyone—and know exactly where to find them.

St. Joe's defined me; it defined us. All these dads coming to
York from all these places to work at all these companies, bring-
ing with them all their families. Some of the dads came to York
ahead of their wives and kids. Mr. McEntee came first. Mrs.
McEntee arrived a few weeks later, her brother driving her
from Peoria to Chicago, where she took the overnight train to
York with three kids in tow. Another dad came by train ahead of
his wife. He got out at the station, looked around and said, "My
God, she's gonna kill me." Mr. Bauler arrived early and then
Mrs. Bauler flew in with two small boys. Riding to York on a

two-lane road cutting between the cornfields and the cow pas-
tures, the young wife who had grown up in Los Angeles looked
around and burst into tears. It was at St. Joe's church and
school where these moms and dads shared this common story
and set about writing a new one together. St. Joe's provided the
rallying point, the haven, where situation and circumstance
converged. Back in those days families didn't go "home" for
Christmas. Who could afford that? No, York was home, it had
to be, right from the start.

================

Once while up in Fairbanks visiting Noreen and me, Mom
paid our group of friends the highest of compliments. She said
it reminded her of the York Crowd. A number of couples
moved from far away to a brand new place, drawn together by
common purpose (in our case the Jesuit Volunteer Corps) and
forced by geography to make a go of it on our own. Indeed,
Fairbanks had always reminded me of York, if bleaker and
colder. Like York, Fairbanks is bordered by a ridge of hills running the full length down one side. Perhaps that is why I liked
it so much, against all the aesthetic odds. The town exists because in 1902 Felix Pedro from Bologna, Italy, discovered gold
on a creek near where a Capt. E.T. Barnette had the year before off-loaded a large cache of supplies he had hoped to get
farther north to start a trading post. Business met opportunity,
or vice versa, and the last of the great gold rushes in North
America was under way.

My Equinox Marathon in September 1982 proved far more
mundane and much less dramatic than Murph's fabulous tri-

umph of 1978, backed as it was by the enthusiasms of brother Billy. My goal was to complete the course in "something that begins with a four." It was merely about finishing, though with a flourish, if I could muster one. It was not to be my first Equinox, even if I considered it such. In 1980, employed as a resident adviser in one of the university dorms, I had rallied the troops to enter the Equinox hiking division. I achieved at least some success, as perhaps eighty of the 200-plus Moore Hall kids showed up at the starting line. (With green stickers reading, "I'm walking 26.2 Moore Miles.") I have no idea how many actually finished. I, needless to say, had to—*had to*—and I did, though well north of nine hours. On the final approach I reached into a mailbox and pulled out a *Fairbanks Daily News-Miner*, the evening newspaper, and read the front page story about the race I was still running. Later, to get out of the bathtub I literally had to inch myself over the side and slide onto the floor, like one of those flabby, lethargic mud suckers that we occasionally hooked into down at Muddy Creek. It took probably fifteen minutes before I could stand up, another fifteen sitting on the side of the bed before I could reach down to put on my socks without toppling over. So "flourish" here was to be a relative term.

As it happened, Noreen and I had arrived in Fairbanks at the beginning of a golden age for the Equinox Marathon. Not because Murph had won. Or not simply because he had won and then won again in 1979. It was because the next year he lost. That newspaper I read to distract me from the awfulness I was feeling talked of someone named Stan Justice, whom none of us had ever heard of, winning in 2:44:59, nearly two and half minutes faster than Murph's record the year before. And with that began a terrific big-time rivalry in what I have never considered a small-time race.

From 1978 to 1994, Murph and Stan won twelve of the sixteen Equinox Marathons run. (The race was officially snowed out in 1992.) Each won six times. Stan's 2:41:30 in 1984 remains the course record; Murph's personal best of 2:46:05, set during his 1980 second place to Stan, would win every race since 1987. Their dominance startles. Murph won his first race at age twenty-six, his last at forty-two, making him the oldest winner. Of the top 100 overall times, they each own 10. In both 1980 (Stan first; Murph second) and 1982 (Murph; Stan) the top five finishers all posted sub-three-hour clockings, the only two times that has happened. Dan Callahan's fifth-place time of 2:56:13 in 1980 would have beat the 2004 winner—by 59 seconds. What NBC wouldn't give to hype this kind of history on its Olympics broadcast.

Of more meaningful importance, Murph and Stan accomplished all this with style and grace. They conducted themselves the way we wish all of our big-time athletes still did. They were old-fashioned, gentleman competitors, their rivalry always just one facet of a larger diamond. The reason I needed to get out of that tub was to get to the "victory" party already planned at Murph's house, which he had immediately redirected as a coronation for Stan. They were both magnanimous in victory, gracious in defeat; it got to where I didn't care who won or lost. Well, almost.

I spent fifteen months preparing for that 1982 Equinox, running through the winter, slowly adding miles. Thirty-mile weeks begat forty, fifty, finally sixty, with a twenty-miler on the weekend. In May I returned to the pipeline corridor where the year before I'd been left for dead (or so I saw it) and ran to the top and over the other side. Not fast by any means (I was never going to be fast), but I did it.

Once, driving south to Fairbanks down the Elliott Highway, I crested a hill. There in the distance—the deep, deep-distance—was Denali, the recently renamed Mount McKinley, the highest point in North America. Living in Alaska, one knows never to take a Denali sighting for granted. The mountain is so colossal, so cold, that it can shroud itself in its own weather even as the rest of the Alaska Range glistens in the sun. From this vantage point it was barely a rock on the horizon at the far edge of a table—if I didn't know where to look I wouldn't have seen it. Still, it was there, as if a giant thumb and forefinger had reached down and crimped the sky right where it meets the earth, creating just hints of shadow and light. I pulled my Honda off the road and reached for my running gear, glad I had thrown a bag in the back that morning. A quick change and I was off on a fifteen-miler. It was August, probably after 10:00 P.M. The sun had only recently set, and the sky was awash in oranges and pinks, courtesy of the severe angle of the northern sun. The area around Fairbanks, the North Star Borough, doesn't lend itself to the Alaska post-card picture. No majestic pine trees, no snow-capped mountains plunging into clear-blue lakes. Just high rolling hills of no breathtaking consequence, stands of stunted pines twisted on themselves by a permafrost that wrecks the roots, birch trees and meandering creeks, any promise of gold long played out. What can overwhelm, if you let it, is to realize that there is so much of it, so much land, too much to see. Denali had to be 150 miles away. Running down to it, I felt like I owned the world.

In those months of Equinox preparation, I embraced the running boom, however tardily. Frank Shorter's victory at the Munich Olympic Marathon had been ten years before. And Bill Rodgers had won the last of his four straight New York City Marathons (another running-boom benchmark) three years prior. But that was the beauty of the Forty-Ninth State in those days, with satellite TV still a newfangled thing. The Last Frontier was not like living in the Lower Forty-Eight. We could do the running boom on our own terms. The New York City Marathon didn't matter; the Equinox did.

For inspiration I read Jim Fixx's "The Complete Book of Running," though it was already five years old. "I ask you to trust me," he writes in chapter five. "The goal, I promise, is worth the struggle." His gospel consumed me. Run, run, always run. Amen. Even when Fixx died of a heart attack barely two years later—while on a run in Vermont—I refused not to believe. Fixx was fifty-two years old. His own father had died of a heart attack at age forty-three (after a first attack at thirty-six). I did the math as others smirked that this disproved what Fixx had espoused. An autopsy showed he had three blocked coronary arteries—one all but completely. He could have done more; he should have done more. But look at what he had done! When he started running, he was some forty pounds overweight and a two-pack-a-day smoker. What he did purchased nine years beyond his father. That's how I figured it then; it's how I figure it now. If my Dad had done that—*if Dad had done that*—he would have lived to sixty-two, shook my hand at my wedding, looked me in the eye, given my bride a kiss. But like Dad quitting the smokes, I can't imagine it. As for me, nine years more gets me to fifty-nine—only three months from sixty, to be exact. Patrick will be twenty-one, with five years of father I never got. For starters, just for starters, I'll take it.

I achieved my Equinox goal of "something beginning with a four": Four hours, fifty-nine minutes, forty-eight seconds. I was ecstatic. I was also unable to move. Once I could finally stop, my legs locked. When Noreen came running up to me I was afraid she was going to tip me over, as if I were a sleeping cow on a dairy farm in York County. I grabbed hold of her, and she held me up until I could move my legs. Murph had won, beating Stan by one minute and twenty seconds. And Pat Kling had won the women's race for the second time, setting another record, in 3:35.52. "P.K.," from Grants Pass, Oregon, had been in the Peace Corps in Brazil and had a sister in the Jesuit Volunteer Corps. Like Murph, P.K. was a grade school teacher. Like Murph, like me, her father had died of a heart attack; he died in 1968. Mr. Kling was fifty; P.K. was twenty-two. She had just begun her Peace Corps commitment. She came home for the funeral then went back. P.K. could run forever. Once, a bunch of us were on a relay team for a charity event from Denali National Park to Fairbanks—a good 120 miles. The second day, P.K. did an 18-mile leg. Another team, from the local

Army base, threw its entire arsenal at her in three- and four-mile bursts. Each soldier got out ahead of her, but she always reeled him in. When she handed off she still had the lead. Quirky, with a kooky sense of humor and a singular laugh—it would often go completely silent, just a look of laughter left on her lips—she was integral to the "Fairbanks Crowd" that Mom had identified. Murph and P.K., winners together.

It was a sweet day. One of the best. More so because two weeks later Noreen and I were gone, driving our Honda back to the East Coast. We had come to Fairbanks on an Equinox victory; four years later we left on another (two more, really). In between, inspired by Murph and tempered not by heat but arctic cold, I became a runner. Standing beyond the finish line of the Equinox, my legs stiff as fence posts, leaning on Noreen, I knew two things. That I would likely never run another one of these again. Not just the Equinox here, but any marathon anywhere. As much as I had enjoyed it—and I loved every mile of it, especially the final quarter I needed to roll to a stop after the finish line—I realized that to attempt it again risked quitting completely. It just did. I cannot fathom how these marathon people line up again and again. But I also realized that I could keep the promise I'd made to me, to Dad (and eventually to Patrick) back on the junior-high track. I now knew I could stay in shape forever. I could do Dad's "road work." I would say that filled me with warm satisfaction, except right then I was trying to get my knees to bend.

Over the years this realization has evolved into the understanding that to stay in good shape I had to let go of the goal of excellent shape. You can't sustain "excellent." At least I can't.

But you can maintain "good." Perhaps that goes as far back as the junior high track. As much as I wanted to be Tommie Smith, American 200-meter gold medalist, I was equally intrigued by the idea of being "just" Peter Norman, Australian silver medalist. Good but not great would be good enough for me.

Running remained for years my preferred method of promise keeping. It was easy, it was cheap; I could do it anywhere. I was probably about thirty-five when—suddenly, as I recall—I switched to every other day. The day after a run on Brooklyn concrete my knees would be screaming. I was no longer a senior in college enjoying my one brief moment as a basketball star, the price exacted the day after games in aching legs that reduced me to tears. That had been worth it, that had been noble. To try to run through it now would have been stupid. I would have quit for sure. So for a few more years it was running, every other day. Though on vacations down the Jersey Shore I would ramp it up to insane levels for the week—ten, eleven miles late in the day, ending with a sprint into the surf—just to see if I still had it. I always did.

Likewise, when friends of a similar running bent visited in Brooklyn, I often took them on running "tours." The bakery around the corner on Henry and Sackett streets where Cher and Nicholas Cage filmed *Moonstruck* was the starting point. Then it was up into Brooklyn Heights past the Hotel Bossert, where the 1955 Brooklyn Dodgers celebrated their lone World Series victory. Mom had lived on Pineapple Street across from the St. George Hotel, where she swam in the Art Deco saltwater pool that looked like a film set for a Busby

Berkeley musical, so we had to go by there next. That with the Dodgers provided an opening for a bit of family lore. In the autumn of 1953 or 1956, when Kathy was either four or seven, the mailman found her wandering outside our house. "My Mommy's crying," Kathy told him. Why, he asked. "Because the Yankees just beat the Dodgers in the World Series."

From there it was down to the Promenade and the stunning view across the East River to Manhattan, then over the wooden walkway of the Brooklyn Bridge, our borough's cathedral, flanked by the gossamer guy lines of the suspension cables. Around City Hall and back again—eight, nine, ten miles total, depending on how much I wanted to show off—talking all the way, a sure sign of shape.

My running life changed forever in September 1988. Noreen and I moved into a new apartment in Brooklyn, a brand-new, too-hip-for-me loft space in an up-and-coming neighborhood. We painted the bare space while watching the Summer Olympics from Seoul, South Korea, on a tiny black-and-white TV. The place came complete with a fitness center in the basement, the fitness center coming with a Concept2 rowing machine. A first-generation model, it had an exposed flywheel and a block of wood for a footrest. Looking back, it was an absolute dinosaur of a thing, ugly and ungainly. And I loved it.

The idea of rowing had long intrigued me. In 1964 the Vesper Boat Club from Philadelphia won the Olympic gold medal as the U.S. eight-oared shell, and the next January some members of that team had come to the York Area Sports Night, a big, big deal on the local calendar. And Dad once bought some sort of at-home rowing contraption—a wooden handle attached by a long, thick spring to a metal-bar footrest, from which extended two rails for a metal seat to slide back and forth. You planted your butt and pushed back with your legs while simultaneously pulling on the handle, which extended the spring. It was all very complicated. It also didn't work. With the handle pulled to your stomach and the spring extended, any slack in the tension and you risked being whipped out of the seat by a suddenly contracting spring. And Dad, ever-cautious Dad, was probably correct when he said that eventually the coil would come loose from the footrest and whack him in the face like a striking cobra.

What I remember best about it, though, is Dad remarking offhandedly that as tall as I was—"rangy," he called it—I would make a good rower.

I took immediately to the machine in the fitness room. I was the only tenant who used the place regularly; it got to when someone else showed up I felt like they had just walked into my own basement. I took Patrick with me, ensconcing him in his car seat next to the rowing machine. Then I made the beginner's mistake of thinking the power of the row is all in the back and shoulders. I was reaching too far forward with the handle, well past my feet and then, from that fully compressed position, yanking for all I was worth. Inside of a month all that enthusiasm had immobilized my neck and shoulders. I was so stiff in the morning that I literally had to put a hand on each side of my jaw to work my head slowly back and forth. And it took me far longer than I care to admit that the problem was me and not the machine.

Soliciting expert advice helped. I was then working at *American Health* magazine, where a contributing editor had been a member of the 1980 U.S. Olympic Eight—the glamour boat—on the ill-fated Olympic team that didn't compete in Moscow because of the U.S. boycott. He offered two pointers. First, let the big muscles of the legs do the work. Second, think of the handle not as a twelve-inch piece of wood but as an oar twenty feet long. My eureka moment. I could plainly see it. I stopped lifting the handle over my knees; doing so digs the "oar" into the water. I was off and rowing. Though not before my Olympic coach offered one final observation: that were I to put my rowing machine in the water, it would sink. As a member of the rowing fraternity's most elite (and elitist) order, he seemed almost required to say this to the likes of me. But I caught his point and still appreciate the advice. It has kept me humble even as I have now rowed, by conservative estimate, some 1,140,000 meters in nineteen years.

The rowing machine provides something near the perfect exercise. It hits virtually all the major muscle groups (except, much to the bad in my case, the pectoral muscles of the chest). But it can be used aerobically for the heart and lungs or anaerobically to build muscle. A rowing machine employs air, not water, against you. The more air resistance dialed in, the more the machine becomes a muscle builder. No surprise, I concentrate on the cardiopulmonary benefits, keeping the air resistance on the fan-wheel dial between three and four (of ten). That allows me to maintain a comfortable 500-meter pace of 2 minutes, 20 seconds, at twenty-three to twenty-four strokes per minute. And I proudly mean "maintain": nineteen years ago when I sat on the sliding seat with no idea what I was doing, that 2:20 pace came to me naturally. I was thirty-eight years old. I'm fifty-five now, but still rowing as fast as ever.

The rowing machine comes as close as possible to putting the lie to the slog of Dad's "road work" dictum. It's not that it's fun. It isn't. It's that I can lose myself so easily in the motion, become the rhythm. The time spent doesn't fly by, it ceases to exist. When I "reach" with the handle in front of me and then "catch" the momentum of the flywheel when I begin to pull back again, that's as perfect a moment as exists in my exercise life. Rowing is the only exercise in which I approach something near the Zenlike state that the fitness gurus advertise, espouse, guarantee. Even then it doesn't come often, but come it does.

Subsequent Concept2 iterations have been designed to make the rowing action easier—a theory I have never grasped. This should be hard, shouldn't it? But the love remains. I could no more now do a "sprint" workout running outside on a track than I could win the 200-meter gold medal at the 1972 Munich Olympics. I'd snap my Achilles' tendon, I'm sure of it. (My fear of snapping an Achilles' tendon far outstrips any heart-attack worry.) I could probably do such a workout on the bike, except I'm too much the wuss to get up to speed. I have been in Brooklyn's Prospect Park minding my business when I've been passed on both sides by a freight train of serious bikers that leaves me gripping the handlebars, unsure if I remember how to steer. No, it's the rowing machine for me.

To maintain this love I play around. I spent one summer swimming at an outdoor pool deep in Red Hook Brooklyn, at a

fabulous brick facility built during the Depression. I learned to
ice skate so I could skate with Patrick, then spent a couple of
winters inscribing ovals at the early-morning adults-only rink
time. For Father's Day in 1991, Noreen bought me a bicycle.
Seventeen months later, on my fortieth birthday, I did my own
Steve McKee Happy Birthday Forty-Forty Biathlon—yes, I
named it—a forty-minute bike followed by a forty-minute run.
I prepared for months, and on the appointed day aged twenty
years. I felt so good I went for sixty minutes each.

I also spent about eighteen months with video aerobics. I
did it only when I was alone in the house. Aerobics got me into
the kind of shape I hadn't been in since college, playing basketball. That had produced an all-around shape of sprinting,
jumping, shooting, backpedaling, sidestepping, and falling on
my butt. So did aerobics. I made my own tape by cadging routines from the early-morning TV fitness shows. Sixty-plus minutes of the not-unmasculine segments with guy instructors
plus a couple of shadow-boxing routines featuring a female instructor with hard Brooklyn accent and thighs so taut they
could have snapped me in half.

Finally, in the winter of 1993-94, I discovered weight training. I was working for a trio of men's exercise magazines that received lots of swag from hopeful equipment manufacturers. The
editor asked me to try one at home—a couple of snap-together
plastic bars with long rubber bands to provide resistance. It
promised a quick and convenient method for taking the gym
anywhere. It delivered a time-consuming and complicated
amalgam of exercises that required too much threading of
bands and resnapping of bars. But it also worked. There was

heavy snow that season, so, with nothing else to do, I did the rubber-band routine. The weather broke in March, and at the first opportunity I got four-year-old Patrick to the playground. As the "older dad" of a toddler, it was always a point of honor that I keep up with my son. Up the ladder, down the slide, hand-over-hand on the bars. Three-quarters through, a much-younger dad walked up and said he was getting tired just watching me. He was right. I wasn't tired, not at all. I joined a health club, for the first time, to hit the weights.

I enjoy resistance training only sort of. It can be time consuming and dull, a task to be done with for the day. That my best efforts have never rendered me even remotely "buff" or "shredded" or "ripped" or "cut" hasn't helped. And I will never have "abs." (I am a huge fan of the long-sleeved T-shirt.) Still, I do it. There is nothing quite like adding more weight to the bar.

I wish now I had started lifting a long, long time ago. York is "Muscletown USA." For three decades—the 1930s, 1940s, and 1950s—a handful of weight lifters who had moved to York to train dominated the national and international "iron game." The tide didn't turn until the 1960s when the Soviets (and anabolic steroids) altered the landscape. I went to school with some of the kids of these men. Their dads were oddly shaped, giant wedges up top funneling down to skinny middles, all of it perched on barrel-like legs. In a double-breasted suit they looked almost cartoonish, as wide shoulder to shoulder as outdoor billboards.

The driving force behind this gang of lifters was Bob Hoffman, a dynamic entrepreneur of large ego who demanded and was accorded a cultlike following. Originally in the oil-burner business, by 1938 he was the majordomo of the York Barbell Company. He coached a couple of Olympic teams, and his club made frequent trips on behalf of the State Department to places like Moscow, Tehran, and Baghdad. He was a huge figure on the local scene for years, a bit of a crackpot to some, espousing the benefits of the physical life well before anyone was willing to listen. Though perhaps Mom and Dad tilted an ear his way. Once when I was in the eighth grade, I was walking around in my underwear at the house, when suddenly they started talking to me about how I was "maturing" nicely and how well my body was "developing." Muscular and defined. Of course, I wasn't and it wasn't. Clearly, they had decided their son's self-image needed some bucking up, and so they had conspired to shower me in compliments. Soon I was posing for them in physique-contest fashion, feeling tremendously good about myself, their goal achieved. Not long after, Dad bought me some York barbells, the classic starter set, the plates sealed in gold plastic. Weight lifting would have done my confidence a world of good at that moment in my life. I regret I didn't grab the opportunity.

=====

Perhaps my favorite run, back before rowing ruled, was my annual eight, nine, ten miler through Haines Acres. That was back in a pre-Patrick world that is difficult now to recall, when Noreen and I would catch the train from Penn Station and go "home" for Christmas. Indeed, before Patrick, York was home, even if I hadn't lived there for nearly twenty years. I'd take off for an hour and a half, two hours and wend my way past the decorated homes of the York Crowd, secure in knowing I could still do the same routine even though another year older.

Most all of them still lived in the Acres then, some from the beginning in 1954, when the development started out with a handful of homes on four blocks off Haines Road. Three bedrooms, one bath, and a carport (an enclosed garage was extra) for perhaps $14,000, the mortgage around 6 percent. There were septic tanks until the sewers were dug and maybe a couple of planks from the front steps to the driveway until the walkways (and, later, sidewalks) were poured.

Sometimes, timing is everything. Haines Acres had it. York welcomed home its veterans from World War II, and like veterans everywhere, they wanted their piece of the American pie. They had *earned* it. York's burgeoning industry was coming East, and people wanted to live close by. And of course then came Caterpillar and all its transferred families, the place open for business in late 1953. Haines Acres to CAT's main entrance turned out to be nine-tenths of a mile.

The Acres were named for Mahlon N. Haines, a wildly successful local shoe-store salesman. Haines was York's "Shoe Wizard" by self-proclamation (he owned about forty shoe stores), an eccentric philanthropist and world-class promoter. In 1948 he built the famous (at least to us) York Shoe House, a clodhopper-shaped, pink cement-stucco thing 25 feet tall, 48 feet long, and 17 feet wide. He provided it free to elderly couples for weekends and to newlyweds for honeymoons, complete with a butler and a maid. For us kids it was a popular destination on summer bike hikes. The Shoe House was ours.

Not a year after I started at the *Wall Street Journal*—well within the I-can't-believe-it stage—the front page of the Marketplace section featured a story about York's Shoe House. I considered that a good omen.

There is more to the naming of Haines Acres. Abraham Epstein, the paterfamilias of Epstein & Sons, Inc., the realty and development company hugely responsible for transforming postwar York, had long had his eye on a very choice 204-acre dairy farm east of York. Owner Haines had always rebuffed his overtures, until one day the two happened to meet downtown. You ever going to sell me that farm? Epstein asked. Yes, blurted the unpredictable Haines, with one predictable proviso: That Epstein names the place "Haines Acres." (It is often called, in York patois, *Haines's* Acres.) Not missing a beat, Epstein said only if Haines made a contribution to a local charity. In March 1954, Haines donated $1,000 to the Girl Scouts, or $2,500 to the Boy Scouts, depending on the story, and Haines Acres had its inevitable sobriquet.

Over about a twenty-five-year period, Haines Acres grew into exactly what it always was, even when the newly planted trees and shrubs were mere sticks poking from the ground: the classic American postwar middle-class white suburban neighborhood. I offer this description without judgment, even as I am now aware of its limitations. Our home on Stanford Drive, built in 1960, was a third-generation Haines Acres offering. An enclosed single-car garage was standard by then, as was a powder room off the foyer and a separate TV room. That reserved the living room for the more formal functions. This was living. Epstein & Sons built the kind of place people wanted to live in, or people wanted to live in the kind of house the Epsteins built. One or the other, and which came first never mattered. They were made of brick and were solidly constructed, even if from an assembly line. Split level (ours), ranch, colonial. The demand was constrained only by the Epstein's ability to procure more land to build on. There was a new iteration of Haines Acres housing under way until well past 1980, as the Realtors continued to buy up the bordering tracts and build homes until they had nearly 800 acres and 1,600 houses. They grew more elaborate as they climbed the hills. Master-bedroom baths, finished basements, two-car garages, custom extensions. Thousands of years from now archeologists will have a field day brushing the dust from these layers of prosperity.

"I don't think your dad ever wanted to move into Haines Acres," Mrs. Schmitt said when I was interviewing in York. Selfish me, I had never thought of that. Never. But she had to be right. Not so much because Haines Acres didn't suit him (though with its closer-together houses and small lots, it likely didn't) but because Wilshire Drive farther east in Stony Brook surely did. It was an already established neighborhood. We had a huge yard, with an additional "back forty." From the kitchen door you could see a stand of trees—"the woods." Dad couldn't hunt them, but at least he could see some country, beckoning to him. The house was small—one bath, no separate TV room—but so what, he could always finish the basement. The place was big enough for him.

It was Kathy and I who were desperate for Haines Acres. Wilshire Hills was on the other side of an area that included the site of the old Camp Security, a prisoner-of-war stockade during the Revolutionary War. Many of the Hessians held there opted to stay in the country at war's end, bolstering the German population. As the crow flies, our Wilshire house was probably no more than two miles from the Acres. To us it was two hundred, two thousand. I don't specifically remember that we badgered our parents to move, but I'm sure we did. I do recall being aware that a move to Haines Acres would indeed be a move up and that it would be saying as much. But to Dad, what Haines Acres probably screamed the loudest was, "Goodbye to Pirate."

Where do I start with Pirate? He was Dad's hunting dog, an English pointer, a Christmas present from Mom in 1961, maybe 1962. Pick of the litter. We went to a farm so Dad could choose the one he wanted from a squirming mass of brown, white, and still-pink new-born puppies climbing over each other to get at their mother. We had always had dogs— "Winkie" the longest and most successful, an all-white mix whose mother was "Blitz," Aunt Evie's German shepherd. But Pirate was different. He was Dad's dog, not mine and Kathy's. No other Dad had his own dog. And he named him, we didn't. "I'm thinking of calling him Pirate," Dad told us earnestly before he had even brought the dog home. "What do you think?" But we knew our job wasn't to think, just listen. "You know the way he has that brown patch on his face covering just the one eye? I think he looks like a pirate." So he did.

The plan was for Dad to train Pirate himself. He bought the books. He talked to anybody who owned one. Pirate was a house dog as a puppy, but Dad made it clear that eventually

Pirate would go outside. He and Pirate, they had work to do. Dad was already penciling out a design for a pen he would build in the back forty. It would come complete with a doghouse with a pullout shelf for a floor that Dad could clean from outside the pen. He was really proud of that innovation. Only now do I realize how much unfettered joy that dog must have brought him. I remember a picture of Dad and Pirate in the back yard. Dad has a cloth tied to some fishing line and he's using a fishing pole to get the cloth out in front of the dog, twitching it, teaching him to point. The smile on Dad's face.

Then Pirate got hit by a car. Really nailed, right in front of the house by a teenager flying down Wilshire Drive. I can hear the screech of tires, the yelp, the continuous, piercing wail. I was in the front yard. Terrified, I ran across the driveway to the other side of the house, looking but not looking, then into the back yard and up to the back forty, but still unable not to hear. By the time I inched my way back to look around the corner of the house, the street was crowded with people, Dad in the middle, the Corvair—I am positive it was a silver-blue Corvair—still parked a bit sideways in the intersection.

Whatever dog Dad was going to train Pirate to be, after the accident he became something altogether different. His broken leg healed well enough—this dog, how he could run!—but Dad was never really able to reach him, settle him down, bring him to heel. He'd take Pirate out to the fields early Saturday morning during hunting season and let him run until he wore himself out, Dad yelling a blue streak. Only then in the afternoon would we see some of what might have been, Dad and Pirate working the fields together, man and dog sharing a certain something that can be a beauty to behold. Pirate could stay on point forever, which was a good thing, because only rarely did he work close up to Dad. Tearing across a field, on the scent, he'd find it and freeze and go stock still all the way out to his tail, everything trembling, sometimes in a contorted, pretzeled position. Then it was up to Dad, with me right behind him, to get to his dog without flushing the bird from too far away.

After he got hit by the car, Pirate turned mean, distrustful, unpredictable. Dad couldn't wear a white shirt around him. Pirate might attack a white shirt, Dad said, surmising that the dog associated pain with the white-suited vet. We learned this the hard way. Aunt Evie and Uncle Tom were visiting not long after Pirate had convalesced and was back in his pen. Dad brought him into the house, still on the leash. In one flying instant Pirate went right for Uncle Tom, in a white T-shirt. A throaty roar and a frighteningly quick leap and Pirate was almost up to Uncle Tom's neck, taking a bite out of the shirt but somehow missing skin completely. Dad yanked and pulled Pirate away, the dog's toenails scraping and clicking on the hardwood floor. But for all that, it is Uncle Tom I remember best. Six-foot-four, thick chested, an Irish cop and a sometime boxer who had cleaned out a bar or two in his day, he had been standing with his hands on his waist when Pirate came in. Afterward, he was still standing exactly the same way. Uncle Tom hadn't even flinched.

When Dad and I drove to the fields, I could sit in the front seat with Pirate between us. No one else could. Again, learned the hard way. Once Dad took Mr. Schmitt hunting with him.

Once. He got in the passenger's seat, and then Dad came around on the driver's side with Pirate on the leash. Dad opened the door and pulled up on the front seat so Pirate could get in the back. The dog did, but then in one growling bound he leapt over the seat and into the front. Mr. Schmitt barely had time to get an arm up. Pirate bit down on him— "good thing I was wearing a coat," Mr. Schmitt says—and didn't let go until Dad grabbed him and pulled him out of the car. Mr. Schmitt blanches even now when telling this story, still searching for its humor. He rode in the back coming and going (it's amazing, really, that he went at all), while Dad drove with one hand and held Pirate by the collar with the other, the dog with the eye patch staring at the intruder in the back seat.

Dad never gave up on Pirate. The story of Mr. Schmitt grew in legend, and Dad and his dog came in for more than a share of good-natured (and not-undeserved) ribbing. *Red, that dog don't hunt!* Dad took it with a smile and a laugh, and then the next Saturday he'd take Pirate to the field, unleash him, and watch him scream away like a banshee, gone until he wore himself out.

Clearly, there was no place in Haines Acres for a dog like Pirate, not that I was concerned about that. We moved when Kathy was a freshman in high school. In only two more years she was driving, and the distance between points on the globe shrank considerably. We could have stayed on Wilshire Drive, had an extension built—there was space enough. Dad gave Pirate to a colleague he knew through Cole Steel. This man lived on a farm north of York where we used to hunt, and I suppose the idea was for Dad to keep coming out. The next hunting

season we did. On the way back home that day, no dog between us, Dad asked me if I thought it was strange to be out
there with Pirate again. I said it was; in fact, it had been extremely unsettling. Dad had even prepped me beforehand, in-
structing me to let his new master be in control, and still it had
caught me unawares. Pirate was a one-man dog if ever there
was one, and now he belonged to a different man. Dad nodded in agreement, pursed his lips the way he could, and raised
his eyebrows in resignation. Because he was driving, he didn't
turn to me. It was like with the sex talks we had only in the car,
on purpose so there'd be no looking at each other. I turned
and peered through the windshield, too. Who knows, maybe
Dad was relieved the dog and the drama were done. He didn't
say anything else, and I don't recall that we ever went back.

But for me, and Kathy, too, Haines Acres was a prayer answered. We moved in August 1964. That gave me a month before school started to try out the neighborhood, to walk down
to the elementary school, to get picked into a baseball game
and then head over to a friend's house for lunch. Living in
Haines Acres also got me into the district where there was
organized Little League the next summer. I was a tall, weak-
hitting first baseman who was good but not real good with
the glove, though just all-around passable enough to fill in anywhere but pitcher or catcher for whoever was on vacation. The
next year I graduated to Senior League, where on the first ball
hit to me in left field of the first practice I ran into the center
fielder and dislocated my right shoulder. That was at the end
of my freshman year of high school, which had started with a

broken left arm in an ill-advised attempt to make the football team.

Haines Acres was my world. To a fault, likely. York, small-town York, didn't escape the turbulence of the 1960s. Race riots in the summer of 1969 brought National Guard tanks to downtown. Not, it should be noted, to Haines Acres. And I wasn't there, anyway. That was our summer in a cabin overlooking the peaceable waters of Lake Skaneateles up in the New York Finger Lakes. The dads came up on weekends, bringing the latest news. A white cop was shot and killed. A few days later a black woman visiting from South Carolina was gunned down. It was ugly and stayed that way through the summer. A trial more than thirty years later into the death of the African-American woman reopened many old wounds and brought national network TV trucks to downtown. No place is uncomplicated. In April 1970 the city sponsored a "Charrette." It was a conscious effort to bring as many parties as possible across all the walks of York's life into the same room, to talk, to plan, to try to move forward. I attended some of the open-forum sessions, fully bursting with the enthusiasm that would land me in St. Mary's, Alaska, in five years. There was lots of finger pointing and too much bloviating, but overall it's fair to say that the Charrette didn't fail and that it wasn't without success. That it happened at all speaks volumes about York.

That I had "missed" the riots, meanwhile, surely speaks volumes about me and my life. Growing up I had no awareness of the York realities that the summer of 1969 laid bare. Haines Acres as fortress and symbol saw to that. Downtown York was

where I went shopping with Mom, at Bear's Department Store
on the York Square. When we were still out on Wilshire Drive
and Dad was home convalescing from his first heart attack, an
African-American man who worked for him at Cole Steel
came to our house. This was unheard of. An awkward frisson
hung in the air as Dad sat in his recliner, wrapped in a blanket
and bathrobe, and the black man—this being 1963 he would
have been a "Negro" or perhaps "colored"—sat on the sofa,
hat in hand, his fingers nervously clutching at the brim. They
barely spoke. Yet I understood there was something significant
occurring here. This man had knocked on our door and Dad
had opened it. But that's close to the sum total of my experience across the divide.

———————

My run through Haines Acres at Christmastime was in its way
my annual homage to that Wednesday morning after Dad
died, when I walked around our house realizing that the York
Crowd had gotten there before us to try to restore some order
to our life. I would make sure to run past everyone's house,
sometimes knocking at a door to say hello and Merry Christmas before running on. I was always glad when someone was
home.

If I wax sentimental about the York Crowd, it is on purpose.
We McKees are deeply indebted to them, grateful for them.
We had already experienced before their capacity to rally in
the tough times. After Dad's first heart attack we got a healthy
dose of it, a just-right mix of serious assistance and irreverent
humor, dolloped out as needed. Nine days after Dad went into

the hospital, Mr. Schmitt presented him with "A 'Big Red' Coloring Book" ("with crayons") to help Dad pass the time. *To John. From some good friends.* Mr. Schmitt photocopied magazine cartoons and then supplied his own captions, each one taking a poke at a particular York Crowd husband or wife. Mom's, for instance, is of a woman (a bit of a battle ax, looking at it now) behind the wheel of a car crushed on top of a motorcycle cop, his arm extended from beneath the pileup handing the incredulous woman a ticket.

> *THIS IS A CAR.*
> *HELEN HAS DRIVEN THIS CAR.*
> *OH HOW SHE DRIVES!*
> *COLOR ME RUSTY.*

That was the idea. There were cartoons for each member of the York Crowd as then constituted. Mr. and Mrs. Flick, Mr. and Mrs. McEntee, Mr. and Mrs. Bauler, Mr. and Mrs. Schmitt. The lampooned characters each wrote a note to Dad on his or her page. I didn't understand most of the jokes, what with the double entendres and inside references to favored alcoholic beverages. One was of a cocktail party with a man dispensing drinks from a gas pump. And it would be many more years before I figured out that Mrs. Bauler must have been quite the number. In her cartoon she is a shapely pony-tailed golfer in quivering "short-shorts." Opposite the tee box a much-admiring man in the gallery holds an APPLAUSE! sign. Mr. Schmitt took his shot at Pirate, too, with a picture of a wolf that Jack London would have cried over.

THIS IS MY DOG.
I CALL HIM PIRATE.
HE IS A HUNTING DOG.
HE HUNTS PEOPLE.
DON'T COLOR HIM—RUN!!

Dad's 1963 heart attack had been my first inkling of this York Crowd ability to weather the storm, but there came more examples. Once, for instance, Amy Flick, her family's youngest at seven years old, fractured her skull on the concrete when she fell backward off the ladder of the high dive at Wisehaven Swim Club, where we all spent our summer afternoons. Amy was a champion swimmer, fully capable in the deep end. I was at the pool that day, and when I saw the crowd gathering by the diving area, I knew it was Amy. That night the York Crowd gathered—to be together, to have a drink, to talk, hope, wait. Amy would be fine, but that wasn't known that night. The word got out to come to McKees. I have no idea how our place got the call. As so often happened, there was no grand plan, it just sprang forth of its own accord.

I reminded Mrs. Flick of that night when I was in York talking to everyone. She nodded in recognition. If there was a secret to this York Crowd thing, she said, this was it, that it wasn't just about the adults getting together to have a good time. Though certainly there had been plenty of that. "All of us," she said, "We were all concerned about everybody else's kids." I know that to be true.

On February 3, 1973, the York Crowd piled into a bus to come see my college basketball team play Messiah College up near Harrisburg. A bus trip was standard procedure for this gang, with the credit likely belonging to Mrs. Masterson, who in particular loved to get the clan on the move. A bus trip to somewhere—anywhere—always found takers, especially if someone's kid was at the end of the road. Everyone arrived at the appointed parking lot with their libation of choice (bus with bathroom being mandatory), ready for a raucously good time, in full-support mode.

For me that night was a double-edged nightmare. I wasn't supposed to go to Allentown College of St. Francis de Sales, the school in Center Valley, Pennsylvania, that was so small, we liked to say, there wasn't a building big enough to hold the full name of the place. I was signed and sealed for Niagara University, where one of Mom's favorite cousins, Jack Reedy, was a biology professor. Then Dad died, and while I still wanted to go away to school—knew I needed to go away to school—Niagara was now too far. Late my senior year Mom asked me about "that St. Francis place in Allentown." As a sophomore two years before I had attended a recruiting pitch at York Catholic, probably because it got me out of a class. I filled out an application, took a placement test, and got accepted. In May, right before I graduated high school, I was in Buffalo for the funeral of my cousin Denny Callaghan, who had been killed in Vietnam. Back at Aunt Marg and Uncle Leo's afterward, Uncle Jack called me aside. He recently had been to a conference at Allentown College of St. Francis de Sales, he said. "You're going to the right school," he told me. "It's going to be the perfect place." And he was right. How so much can turn on so little.

Allentown College of St. Francis de Sales was a brand new school, rising literally from the cornfields, the place making itself up as it went along. When I arrived in the fall of 1970 there had been only two graduating classes. The school's only real resource was the students themselves, maybe 400 total, and the Oblates of St. Francis de Sales tapped into us, asking for everything we had. A fledgling theater program was the school's calling card then, but there was also a basketball program taking its first baby steps beyond the club level into varsity status. Back at York Catholic I had been cut from the basketball team my sophomore year, terrified of running my tall, skinny self onto the court in gold-and-green underwear. When Jim Forjan, York Catholic's basketball coach, rescued me my senior year, taking me into his office and under his wing for seventh-period study hall, I regretted immensely that I had never tried again. The Centaurs of Allentown College, their level of play dovetailing nicely with my nascent talent, offered me a chance at redemption in red and blue. And on this night, with the York Crowd as witness, at no less of a place than Messiah.

I was a junior by then, already a two-year starter. But I had recently lost my first-five spot, so with my own private cheering section having arrived primed and in plenty of time, the game began without me. Messiah was one of three Christian liberal arts colleges we played every season. "Bible schools," to us Catholics, they played a ferociously disciplined game, all crisp fundamentals, Messiah the best of the lot. They were on their way to a twenty-five-and-seven season; we Centaurs, arriving on an eight-game losing streak, to six-and-eleven. Still, we stayed with them early. With three minutes left in the first half we were down only two before they ran to an eleven-point half-time lead. I played sparingly in the first twenty, at one point anxiously launching a shot off the top of the backboard and out of bounds.

The second half "was one disaster after another," as I wrote in a diary I devoted to that dismal season. With barely eight minutes gone the game was completely out of hand, Messiah on the way to a twenty-nine-point pasting, 76–47. This meant that Steve McKee, second-stringer, was now on the court, though not the least bit sure he wanted to be. But then Messiah finally took a notch or two off its crushing intensity. That allowed me to find some space between myself and the guy guarding me, and I proceeded to hit three long jumpers in a row, beautiful rainbows, deep on the left wing—right in front of my bussed-in fans. I knew that the ball was in the basket before it left my fingertips, that the York Crowd behind me was about to roar. We scored twenty points in the second half, and I had eight of them. Soon enough the York Crowd was yelling to get McKee the ball and grumbling loudly about why wasn't he in there when it mattered. I finished with ten points total and eleven rebounds in eighteen minutes.

Mom waited for me outside the locker room after the game. The crowd was back on the bus, ready to go. She asked me to walk her back to say hello. Climbing onto that bus that night was the last thing in the world I wanted to do. The game had been horrifying, a complete embarrassment. *Twenty-nine points.* How could playing for this team—not even starting!— prove that I should have played at York Catholic? But it was also the only thing I wanted to do. I'd gone five for six, really stroked it, doubled my woeful five-points-per-game average. In the score book at least, it would be the best game I played that season. And I knew what awaited me on that bus, and I longed for it. "They don't care about winning or losing," Mom said as I continued to feign reluctance. "They only care about you." I climbed aboard and into a forty-seat, standing-bus ovation.

They were all there that night, all the usual York Crowd suspects. Weren't they always? On that bus; in our house that morning after. They have never not been there. That first Christmas after Dad, we went to dinner Christmas Eve at McEntees, with the Schmitts. Christmas Eve had always been Dad's big moment to celebrate Mom's birthday. Restaurant, gifts, "I'll Never Smile Again." Soon after we returned to our house, Mr. and Mrs. Flick, Philbin, and Masterson announced themselves, barging in, bearing birthday presents. The next morning it was breakfast with the Flicks and Ochses and then dinner at the Philbins, where it was always fun to look out the living room window at all the Christmas lights festooning York. I could go on and on. But perhaps the truest measure here is that it hasn't been only the obvious times, the major moments, when the York Crowd has come through—for Kathy and me whenever we have asked, and for Mom always. No, real proof is in the details. The York Crowd was *young* when Dad died. A fact that becomes more plainly evident the longer they continue to hold on, most of them now into their mid-eighties. Almost everyone has given up smoking. It's amazing, really, that so many of them are still with us. Right from the start they made sure that Mom remained part of the crowd.

Couple club—*couple* club—had always been a significant social night for the York Crowd. A once-a-month card party, rotated from house to house among four or six couples. Dinner, bridge, dessert. After Dad died they solved any fifth-wheel awkwardness by keeping Mom, inviting another couple, and declaring a nonplaying host. Simple. A small example, but that's why it's perfect. Aunt Evie marveled every time she came to visit, forever telling Mom that this wasn't the way it worked. That when a woman's husband died, her life died with him. The York Crowd would have none of that.

I won't pretend that this group of people is one big happy. It isn't; they aren't. They have been friends far too long, and everyone knows each other far too well for that. There have been feuds and spats, and not all of them have been rubbed smooth by time. They are not all everybody's best friends. And if I could gain any distance, I would probably see they are clannish and insular. Yet the York Crowd endures. Mom is as much in the mix now as when it was she and Dad together, charter members. I assume, I hope there are communities of friends like this everywhere. But I don't know that. I do know that everyone should be lucky enough to experience it. Fifty years ago, who knew a white-bread suburban neighborhood—the very kind that is so easy to lampoon—would produce such power, such staying power?

When Patrick came to Noreen and me in 1990, I called Mom to tell her the good news. We were exploding with joy. But there was a synapse missing in her response. I could sense she was trying to meet my happiness in equal measure, but she couldn't. Finally she told me. The husband of a York Crowd kid had been killed in an accident, sustaining catastrophic head injuries. He had been on life support for a few days until the questions of when to remove him and whether to donate organs could be sorted through.

It had all been horrible. This York Crowd kid was one of the youngest. Dad had adored her; she was the apple of his eye. The old days were far removed if this woman-kid could be a widow with two young children.

Our new McKee family flew home to Brooklyn a day early so I could attend the funeral in Pennsylvania. There, I was caught in an awkward swirl of emotions. We had found our son, but she had lost her husband. I hadn't brought a picture, on purpose, but at the luncheon after the cemetery I was roundly chastised for that by the York Crowd, in full presence. I had no idea what to say to anyone. It was her father who rescued me. Kathy always used to say he looked like Lorne Green—Ben Cartwright from Sunday night's *Bonanza*, with his white hair and broad, gentle face. But now here he was, his jowls pulled to the floor by grief and exhaustion. He walked over and threw an arm around me. He had done something much the same once a long time ago as my Confirmation sponsor. Now he seemed to do it just to hold himself up. We stood together in silence. Then finally he spoke. "Steve," he said, "He took one away but He gave us one back."

There it was: the one place where we could stand together and still appreciate each other's opposite moment. "Us," of course, was the York Crowd.

TUESDAY,
SEPTEMBER 30; 10:21 P.M.

Run, steve, run. dad was dead, that's for sure. i knew it even if the cop wouldn't say so. I needed to get to Mom, down at Schmitts playing cards with the moms. I had just gotten my license, and Dad's Chevy was out front, but that wasn't an automatic. He had wanted me to learn on a stick but I'd chickened out. Besides, the keys were probably in his pocket. *Uh-uh.* But how far away could Schmitts be, anyway? Half-mile, tops? Two laps of the junior high track, just one set—walk a 220, jog a 220, run a 220, sprint a 220. I could do that easy, even in school shoes, my black-and-brown saddles. I'd done most of it before. A couple of years ago I stayed overnight at Schmitts, with Mom and Dad away for a weekend. It was the middle of winter, and we'd been outside playing in the snow, roaming all over Haines Acres. By the end of the day my hands were blocks of ice. I ran back to Schmitts, wanting Mom and Dad but knowing Mr. and Mrs. would take care of me. So once the cop radioed for the ambulance there was no reason to stick around. I mean Dad was dead. I dropped his wrist and took off, out the door.

Straight down the Stanford hill, left on Raleigh, first right onto Sundale Drive. If Haines Acres were the human heart— and to me in so many ways it was—then Sundale was its main artery. Flowing down the hill from the top of Eastwood Drive, it ran the length of the development. Now I was, too, pacing myself. Get out too fast and I'd have to walk and that would take too long.

Today, at fifty-five, I could make that half-mile run in a pleasant six minutes, my heart rate a solid 125 beats per. Who knows how long it took that night, or what my heart was up to. Sundale slides down a bit from Raleigh Drive then angles up slightly at Schoolhouse Lane, cresting the drawn-out rise right at Schmitts, on the left. I could see their house most of the way, the porch light on, across the street from the old Haines homestead with its big white barn.

I knew their door wouldn't be locked, and I knew I didn't have to knock. I ran up the driveway and took the steps up to the porch in one bound. Like the time when Kathy was in seventh grade and she'd finished second in the Catholic grade-school spelling bee. We stopped at Schmitts afterward and I burst in the house with the news. Now, I pulled out the screen door and pushed in on the wooden door, exploding right into the living room, where I came to a dead stop. Mom and Mrs. Schmitt, Mrs. Anderson, and Mrs. Malloy were at a card table in the middle of the room. Mr. Schmitt sat at the dining room table. They all looked at me. I looked at them, the exertion of the past few minutes suddenly making me gasp. I had been so intent on running down here that I hadn't thought at all about what to do, what to say, once I did. For a second no one moved. Then I motioned for Mom. "Come here, Mom, come here!"

——————

If running my junior year in high school never got me to the Munich Olympics in 1972, it did get me down to Schmitts that September night in 1969. Thirty-six years later, all my running and biking and rowing (and swimming, ice skating, aerobicizing, and weight lifting) from that night forward is what got me to the Princeton Longevity Center in New Jersey for the day-long physical that revealed my heart disease. That is a conclusion I eventually reached gladly, but certainly not on that day in April 2005 when I sat in Dr. David Fein's office and watched him point on the computer screen to the calcium deposits in my left anterior descending and right coronary arteries and the serious heart disease it suggested.

It hadn't been my idea, this eight-hour "executive physical." Noreen had arranged it and I went along. What could it possibly tell me except that I was in great shape? I know that now to be hubris, but at the time it was just a matter of fact.

Executive physicals have been around for a while, but as their name implies, the original target audience was fairly narrow. Perhaps because these *uber*-checkups aren't cheap (mine was $2,000 plus) and insurance coverage can be spotty. Recent advances in technology have helped to close the cost gap somewhat and, perhaps more important, helped to bring these tests under one roof, seriously upping the convenience factor. Specifics vary, but in general an executive physical offers some form of extra-comprehensive blood testing, nutritional counseling, a stress test, a hearing and lung check, and noninvasive whiz-bang body imaging. Of equal or greater value, you get time with the doctor.

From the outside, the PLC could be just another real-estate office somewhere along New Jersey's Route One corridor. Inside, the place is gleaming and efficient. Everyone speaks in hushed tones. There is almost no one there. The PLC sees only a few patients a day.

Noreen and I arrived at 8:00 A.M., dressed for a workout, me in my favored old-school Green Bay Packers hooded sweatshirt and baggy gray sweat pants. I started with the nutritional analysis. I had submitted beforehand a diary of everything I had eaten for three days. For breakfast, some combination of cinnamon-raisin bagels with a vegetable spread containing plant stanols and/or some shredded wheat sprinkled with a bran cereal with added psyllium. The stanols and the psyllium were a fairly new addition, so perhaps I was cheating to include them. Two years before at a regular physical the doctor said my cholesterol was beginning to inch above 220, pushing the ceiling of acceptable. He had also, based on my EKG and sub-60 resting heart rate and a conversation on what all I was up to, declared me the healthiest fifty-year-old who had ever walked into his office. But with my cholesterol creeping he had wanted to put me on a statin. I resisted mightily and told him, out loud, in a word, NO. I hadn't spent a lifetime staying in shape just to throw it all over to some Godzilla drug company. They were doing just fine without my $15 co-pay. And side effects? Liver problems? Muscle aches? *Muscle damage?* Those were the serious and usually rare side effects, with the dose often critical to the outcome, but there were still the headache, nausea, vomiting, constipation, diarrhea to consider. But mostly, popping some pill wasn't the promise I had made to Dad, to me, to Patrick. I could beat this on my own. For me, for them. That part I said to myself. From the doctor's office I went immediately to a bookstore, where I shopped the self-help shelves, settling on a tome for reducing cholesterol "naturally." Turned out I was already onboard with most of the recommendations, and I was full enough of my own self, thank you very much, to take all the credit.

Back in the mid-1980s I had embraced the then-current heart-healthy diet. We all know the drill here—low fat, complex carbohydrates, etc., etc. I grabbed hold with both hands and wrestled it to the ground. Within months, without trying to or particularly wanting to, I had lost twenty pounds. Friends whom I hadn't seen in a while remarked upon it. I needed to poke new holes in my belt to keep my pants from falling down. I took this diet on for no particular reason beyond the idea that it seemed the next logical step in my stay-in-shape promise. A check of my cholesterol and I had it down below 160. The problem, as with any diet *extremis*, was that its reality was in direct opposition to its practical applicability. It was crazy, in truth, with no foundation in the real world. Steamed fish, skinless chicken, plain baked potatoes. There was more to it than that, but it didn't taste like it. If I will never understand why people smoke, I fully get it when it comes to diet and how enormously difficult one can be. I have come to appreciate that it is better to be on a "good" diet than to be constantly failing to be on a great one. I never officially abandoned my regimen, I just reached a point a few years later when I realized I was no longer on it. But I have ever since adhered to its basic tenets. I was comfortable with the accommodations I had made.

The book on cholesterol lowering did, however, offer up the stanols and psyllium. So I went after both. Plant stanol esters or plant sterols are found in a wide variety of plants and vegetables. They help lower total cholesterol levels and LDL, the notorious "bad" cholesterol, by blocking their absorption. Psyllium is a soluble fiber, a laxative that serves to quicken the digestive process. It, too, works to lower LDL levels and cholesterol absorption. The nutritionists told me to stay with them. With everything else I was doing—the "as part of a diet low in saturated fats and cholesterol" caveat—they could perform as advertised.

Overall in the food analysis I was just a few points shy of the "excellent" score for the low-fat-meal category, and I earned extra points for not skipping breakfast. I was even getting enough fiber. The nutritionist's recommendations were to eat more almonds (fatty, but of the heart-healthy monounsaturated kind) and turn some of the fruit juices into actual fruit (too much juice can lead to too many triglycerides). One more thing, she said: Eat your vegetables.

Next was the treadmill test to assess cardiac function, my overall fitness. If I had arrived in the morning without enthusiasm, I got religion once the EKG leads were stuck all over me. The stress test has been around for about fifty years, but I remembered it best from the Mercury Seven astronaut days. The pictures in *LIFE* magazine of Alan Shepard, Wally Schirra, Gordon Cooper, and all the rest, hooked up to confirm their fitness to be blasted into space to battle the Commies. It was all very, very important stuff.

I stepped on. This test is not infallible. It won't tell you if you have an artery that is, say, "only" 50 percent blocked. But for me, this was it: my life to this moment. I knew I was not in exceptional shape. I was just in the kind of shape I had kept myself in for most of my life. That was always the point, wasn't it? It was time to learn what that shape was. I could feel my heart within me, hear it talking to me. *Let's go.*

I was told I could stay on for a maximum of twenty-five minutes, the speed and the incline slowly increasing. I stepped off at twenty. My maximum heart rate was 169 beats per minute, 101 percent of the predicted rate for my age group. I was an engine. A minute later my heart rate was down to 144; two minutes, 128; five minutes, 108. (The heart's fitness correlates to how quickly the rate descends.) I had the aerobic capacity of a man almost eight years younger; the recovery rate of a man twenty years younger. My "normal," according to the printout, was their "excellent."

The stress test put me in the 86th percentile for men my age. I reached the 90th percentile ("excellent") in trunk flexion; the 70th ("good") in crunch assessment: "perfect muscle firing pattern—47 reps in 1 minute." My upper body strength flat-lined in the 5th percentile after I completed all of two pushups. That was no shocker. I am woeful on the upper body. I once went wave running with Noreen's nephew on the bay at Ocean City, New Jersey. That was perhaps twenty years ago, and we were on first-generation machines. You had to hold on to the handlebars and lie flat, your legs dangling behind you in the water. After you hit the gas and got some speed, the idea was to punch it again and use that momentum to pop yourself up onto your knees. The twelve-year-old nephew punched, popped, and was gone. I punched, but I could never pop. The machine would get away from me, and I'd tread water while it circled around and came back, as designed. I was in a bad *Jaws* remake, the machine slowly stalking me. Finally, near exhaustion, I gave up. I conceded that drowning was a worse option than humiliation, if only just. I held on and let the machine drag me back to the dock, where the next group gawked, the exhaust from the machine filling my swimsuit before bubbling out the pant legs.

That 5th percentile pulled down my Overall Fitness Score to 81. I didn't care. I was thrilled. If 90-plus would have gotten me gold, 80-plus was solid silver. For all these years, hadn't that been the idea? The next assignment was the interview with the doctor. I told him my story gleefully. A scan to take a series of pictures of my heart and then a full-body scan for a final look-see and to check for osteoporosis rounded out the day. All that remained was the final consult with the doctor at day's end. I was still in my sweats, dressed for the victory stand, ready for my lifetime-achievement award.

Noreen told me later that when I came out of Dr. Fein's office she knew immediately that the news was not good. But I must applaud him. He was terrific. He wears bold-colored shirts and bold-checked ties. He has a bold, irreverent sense of humor that I found hard to resist. And he believes in his business. He is, he said, in a way merely in data collection. Knowledge was everything.

When I sat down he started talking immediately, chatting up all the good news. Great shape, right track on the diet, all that. And then—seamlessly, effortlessly—he turned my attention to the computer screen on his desk. He explained the technology that permitted us to take the heart and slice it into so many separate slides across an entire cross-section of the organ.

He turned the screen so I could see it. There were shapes in various shades of black and gray. It took me awhile to get oriented—breastbone up, backbone down. He clicked back and forth between the first three or four pictures so I could see how one slide morphed into another and then another. Finally it came alive. With that he started, and together we looked into my heart.

He did such a good job with his explanations that when I saw it he didn't have to say a word. After a couple of images in blacks and grays, suddenly there appeared a line of white—a milky, bony, old man's finger, the Ghost of Christmas Future clutching at my heart. The doctor clicked a few more times and it grew in length and thickness, eventually through about 20 percent of my left anterior descending artery. A few more clicks, and there was more of the same in my right coronary artery. The white indicated the presence of calcium, he said, which in turn suggested the presence of plaque in my arteries. He ran through the calcium scorecard. A reading of one to ten is considered a "minimal" score; 11 to 100, "mild"; 101 to 400, "moderate"; over 400, "severe." I had clocked in at 452. My cholesterol stood at 266, at least 60 points too high; my triglycerides were at 315, more than double a good reading. Given my calcium score, the doctor said, my risk that day of a heart attack in the next twelve months was

10 percent. If left untreated there would be no "risk." A heart attack would become a certainty.

My throat tightened, my lips trembled. Unable to speak, I held up my hands—to surrender to him, to beg him to stop. Please. Dr. Fein has become a great ally in all this. But not that day. The junior high track. The Equinox. The rowing machine. All I could do was shake my head slowly from side to side. The numbers added up to the sum of all fears.

━━━━━━

"Dad's dead, Mom! Dad's dead!" I didn't wait for her to walk over to me at the Schmitts' door. I lunged and threw my arms around her. She recoiled. Between my gulps for air and gasps of my crying, she clearly didn't understand what I was saying, but just as clearly she knew it had to be awful. Years later she told me she heard "Dad's *drun*k," and that had made no sense at all. It was 10:30 on a Tuesday night, and she'd been gone less than three hours.

I don't remember what else I told them, aside from the fact that Dad was dead. Did I use the words "heart attack"? Surely I had put it all together already. I had seen it, after all. And hadn't we been waiting for this other shoe to drop, another artery to clot? Now it had, and Dad was dead, for sure.

Mr. Schmitt took over. Mrs. Schmitt and the other moms would wait here for a phone call. He'd go with Mom and me to the house. I tried to tell him Dad was dead. He kept me moving outside. At Mom's car out front, I tried one more time. I was around the driver's side; Mr. Schmitt was going to drive but he was opening the door for Mom. I leaned my arms on the vinyl roof. "Dad's dead! Dad's dead!" I blurted it out, desperate to be heard, spreading my arms across the roof of the car for support. "Steve," this was Mr. Schmitt, stern and no-nonsense. "Get in the car. Get. In. The. Car." His voice slapped my face. I got in the car. Mr. Schmitt came around, and silently we drove back up Sundale, then left on Raleigh. A short block on the right and it was immediately up the steep hill of Stanford. Our house was up on the left, distinguishable from the others only by the black plastic American eagle Dad had nailed to the brick over the front door. It sounds tacky, but from the street it had a solid, permanent, people-live-here look. The ambulance was backed in our driveway, its blinking red lights bouncing off the garage doors of the other houses. I didn't go in. Mom and Mr. Schmitt did, but they were back out only moments later behind Dad, strapped and lifeless on the gurney.

Mom doesn't remember if she called for an ambulance or drove Dad to the hospital when he had his first attack. This time she either rode with Dad or Mr. Schmitt took her, but again she doesn't remember, and neither do I or Mr. Schmitt. I got dropped at Schmitts, and he followed the ambulance. The plan now was for Mr. Schmitt to call as soon as he had something to report. So we waited, Mrs. Schmitt and me. Jimmy Schmitt was a senior at York Catholic with me, and there were also Kathy, Chrissie, Steve, John, and Greg. This was a school night and they had to be there—but for me the house was empty save for the presence of Mrs. Schmitt, who kept up a hopeful chatter. Then the phone rang. It was time to go.

Mrs. Schmitt maintained the optimistic banter on the drive across town to York Hospital. She particularly thought that having a cop drive by at the precise moment I was running back to our house after trying to get a neighbor to help had to be a good sign. Very good. What were the chances? This was Haines Acres, where the cops didn't cruise the streets, yet there he was. I listened to everything, trying to believe, wanting to believe. But I already knew. Dad was dead. I had seen it. Hadn't they heard me tell them so?

York Hospital is maybe three miles from Haines Acres. Mount Rose Avenue to Boundary Avenue, Boundary to Vander Street and past York Catholic, Rathton Road across Queen Street and there it was. I knew the route too well, having traversed it nearly every day for too many weeks six years before. In 1969, York Hospital's emergency entrance was next door to the main entrance, so we drove straight in the main driveway and up the hill. Mr. Schmitt saw the car. He left Mom and started walking toward us. When I got out he pointed behind him. "You need to go over to your mother." She was standing by our Cutlass, alone and lost, arms folded in front of her, her lips gone thin, her jaw set.

I walked over and tried to put my arms around her, the way I had always seen Dad do it. Though Mom was 5-foot-8, Dad, at about 6-foot-1, would always sort of bend at the knees a little bit rather than at the waist when giving Mom a hug, maybe because his back was always in danger of going out, or maybe because that's how they fit together best. They weren't big huggers, Mom and Dad, but it wasn't unusual, either. When Dad got home from one of his rare business trips, he'd put his suitcase down with one hand and the paper bag in the other that Kathy and I knew held our "Dad's home" presents, and we'd have to wait until the two of them had a nice, long hug. I also see them in the kitchen at Stanford Drive, wrapped together in a bear hug for no reason at all, making this recall all the sweeter. Now, since I was nearly six inches taller than Dad, I was going to need to bend even more at the knees. I tried my best imitation of him, but with my arms not even around her yet, Mom twisted away and climbed into the passenger-side seat. Mr. Schmitt was still down by the emergency entrance. I turned and walked over to the lip of the parking lot, high on the edge of the hill overlooking York out to the west. My hands in my pockets, I stared at the lights until Mr. Schmitt called to me that it was time to go.

═══════

For one final time, Dad was an Everyman for his generation. He died in 1969—just one year after the death rate from heart disease had reached its peak. Not that anyone knew that then. Mom requested an autopsy. For the previous month or so Dad had been experiencing severe, sharp pains in the middle of his back. They sliced at him in such a way that to find relief he had to sit down and arch his back grotesquely, his elbows thrown back as far as he could get them, holding that position for as long as it took to get rid of them. Kathy says Mom's thinking was that perhaps an autopsy could connect a few more of the dots, maybe to these pains.

I have been unable to locate a copy of that autopsy. By official nomenclature Dad died a "natural death," records of which eventually can be destroyed. So we are left with the words on the death certificate, apparently gleaned from the autopsy. TIME OF DEATH: "10:20 P.M." IMMEDIATE CAUSE: "Post right coronary occlusion." INTERVAL BETWEEN ONSET AND DEATH: "Minutes." While I appreciate both its brevity and bluntness, it states the known. The unknown remains.

In the Sherlock Holmes story "The Hound of the Baskervilles," Sir Arthur Conan Doyle describes a man's death as resulting from "cardiac exhaustion," with the man rendered largely unrecognizable by the befalling event. There remains for me something of this in Dad's last night, in what I witnessed when his heart attacked him. "[H]is features convulsed with some strong emotion to such an extent," says an agitated client to Holmes, "that I could hardly have sworn to his identity."

Herewith follows my attempt to swear to Dad's identity, and to the events of his death. To try to know what can't be known. I have talked with a dozen doctors—cardiac physicians and surgeons, emergency-room attendants, pathologists, coroners—and one administrator of a hospital coronary-care unit, asking them to "diagnose" Dad's death. I provided a complete workup. The first attack in 1963; the three packs a day; the fishing episode with Mr. Ochs, when Dad could barely get up the hill; Cole Steel; eggs for breakfast; the back pain; the final Tuesday night. I granted these doctors anonymity in exchange for their opinion on a patient not theirs, dead now nearly forty years. What took place became not a diagnosis but a dialogue, these doctors talking not to me but to each other, complete with contradictions and disagreements. What they say here is not definitive. It is not meant to be. It can't be. But I swear by it.

We're living a lot longer than we were probably designed to. We were designed to live long enough to reproduce. Once we reproduce, the world we live in really has no use for us anymore. We're excess baggage. Our DNA wants us dead.

It all happens very, very fast, . . . because the heart's livelihood depends on that constant supply of oxygen. It's not like it can rest. It has to keep beating during this period when it's getting no oxygen. That's why it happens so incredibly fast. If the heart could say, "I'm going to rest for ten minutes, I'm going to stop while you finish your heart attack . . .," but that doesn't happen. It has to keep going. Meanwhile, there is a growing area that isn't getting oxygen. So more and more cells are dying. There is no downtime for the heart. Even when the oxygen supply is being cut off by that coronary occlusion, it has to keep pumping.

———

What is very significant was the event when he was fishing.

The back pain, I don't think this was angina. I think it more likely to be pericarditis, the inflammation of the lining around the heart. That he could relieve it by finding a certain position is not consistent with heart disease, but it is consistent with pericarditis. He very well might have had a heart attack during the fishing trip, and [the back pain] was post-heart-attack pericarditis.

His heart was probably exhausted, and it wasn't pumping well. Or he was having an arrhythmic bout. The cardiac conduction system wasn't functioning. . . . There might have been a partial clot. The clot formed and then probably dissolved by itself. . . . At some point flow was restored. The heartbeat was re-established to the point that he felt comfortable enough to have a smoke after. Especially if it scared him. The fishing trip definitely seems like . . . a first shot across the bow that said something here is wrong.

─────

[The night he died] he had a sudden occlusion, which gave him a rhythm abnormality, which dropped his blood pressure and gave him what looked like a seizure, but it wasn't.

Usually with the right coronary occlusion, the heart rate becomes very slow, the blood pressure drops, you get a lack of blood flow to the brain, and the patient often has a seizure.

*The arched back and being snapped back and forth?
That's a seizure. You don't get that just from the agony of
how much your chest hurts.*

*The fact that the heart was no longer an efficient pump
meant he wasn't getting oxygen to his brain and that triggered seizures. [It] would've happened very, very quickly.*

*He had no blood flow. His brain quit working. What you
may have been seeing were just neuromuscular reflexes. . . .
The time frame between going into arrhythmia and having a neurological event is just a matter of seconds. That
fits your time frame.*

———

*He was clearly having a lot of pain. He may not have
been able to express it. He wasn't able to say, "Hey, I'm
having a lot of pain here!" It just hurt so much. But it
sounds like it was all over in a matter of seconds.*

*The blessing is you're rendered unconscious pretty
quickly. But he probably did feel some pain.*

*There are people who are having such severe pain that
they have no reaction to it. It is that severe. [And in] a
heart attack, the pain can be that severe.*

*When oxygen gets cut off from the brain there is still about
thirty seconds of consciousness, or semiconsciousness. He*

probably suffered severely for those few seconds. I have to imagine that.

━━━━━━

He had foam coming out of his mouth? He could have gone into pulmonary edema, congestion of the lungs. Because of the extent of the damage [to his heart] there was acute heart failure. And that led to fluid buildup in his lungs.

When the heart fails, fluid backs up into the lungs and it's often kind of frothy. Oxygen has to get into the bloodstream. In exchange, carbon dioxide goes out from the blood into the air sac. There's a delicate equilibrium. If you build up the pressure in the bloodstream, the fluid that's contained in the bloodstream can leak into the air sacs. It's pure physics. If blood vessels don't rupture [from the pressure] then the red blood cells are held in the lung and just the plasma leaks out, and it mixes with air and becomes frothy. Sometimes it's pink if the pressure is high. If larger vessels rupture, or enough rupture, then it can actually be bloody. But more often than not, it's white. A brilliant white.

━━━━━━

It doesn't sound like a classic heart attack to me. The issue of an aortic dissection pops into my head. . . . The arching of the back and all that. . . .

The aorta is the main tube carrying blood around the heart. It's like an old-fashioned tire with layers that go one way and then go the other way. If there is hardening of the arteries, you get a little divot, a small hole. It's damaged and then it gets repaired. It's like a 24/7 road crew. But it gets to the point where the damage crew is making more problems than the repair crew can fix. So this little pothole in the artery expands. High blood pressure forces blood into the pothole, and it can get inside those layers. A layer lifts up, and that's called a dissection. What happens is the rip spirals because these layers are at different angles. Imagine a corkscrew ripping right through it. It disrupts everything and [can] go forward or backward. Forward is an aortic dissection. When you have a backward dissection and it spirals backward, the right coronary artery is commonly associated with it.

In an aortic dissection, people who survive it describe it as "someone ripping my chest apart." They say they can feel the ripping and the tearing. "There was a tearing in my body." "I was being pulled apart."

I don't think the coroner could have missed a dissection. When the coroner opened him up he would have found his chest cavity filled with blood.

If it was the abdominal portion of the aorta, then there wouldn't have been blood in the chest. The blood would have all been stuck in the abdomen. And they wouldn't have seen it, even if they had opened up his chest.

They would have seen that the aorta was violated and discolored. It's an autopsy finding that just jumps out at you. I'm still putting my dollars on acute coronary syndrome.

―――――

If you had the full autopsy report, you might find that there were multiple arteries blocked. . . . It could have been more than one thing going on. . . . The question is whether he had [heart] disease in other arteries.

I say the left anterior descending. "The Widow Maker." That is a very difficult heart attack to survive. Mortality rates are real high on that.

Right coronary occlusion? I assume they mean a real occlusion, and not a partial, which wouldn't be an occlusion but an "obstruction." You can actually lose quite a bit of your right coronary and still have a functioning heart because of collateral [blood] flow. I've done autopsies with just about complete occlusion of the right coronary artery, and it's not what they died of.

Ninety percent of the time the dominant artery—the artery that supplies the heart with the majority of its blood—is on the left side. Ten percent of the time, roughly, the dominant artery is on the right. If the right coronary [was] dominant, and if he lost that artery, he could lose the blood supply to two-thirds of his heart.

The right coronary artery feeds the sinoatrial node, which is the place that starts the heartbeat within the heart. It's the pacemaker for the heart. When it isn't getting enough blood, then that pacing function is lost.

He obviously had extensive coronary artery disease. He ruptured plaque. Vulnerable, high-risk plaque ruptured suddenly, and that led to sudden coronary death. . . .

A nonobstructive plaque ruptured, and he went from 30 or 40 percent blockage [in an artery] to 100 percent in no time flat. . . .

Most heart attacks happen in arteries that are less than 50 percent blocked. It's because of the rupture of that plaque, when the plaque splits open and exposes the inside of that plaque to the blood flow and it forms a clot.

What's going to kill . . . is what we call soft plaque, vulnerable plaque; deposits of cholesterol in the wall of the arteries. [It's] like a little pimple, a cholesterol pimple. One of those pimples burst . . . and [a clot forms] and it causes the sudden cessation of blood flow.

It is still amazing to me that our entire survival is based on our blood going through a pipe that at certain points is less than a centimeter.

The platelets do their job, which is to form a blood clot. They receive the signal that this is an area that needs to be clotted off. It's the same mechanism when you cut yourself shaving. [The problem is that] platelets weren't designed with the idea that they would be faced with people getting plaque in their arteries.

Think of [the platelets as] developing more for stopping the bleeding after we've been attacked by a dinosaur. Platelets were much more important for keeping us from bleeding to death rather than keeping our coronary arteries open.

Inflammation plays a big role in heart attacks. The more inflammation that is present inside the plaque, the greater the likelihood the plaque will rupture—and that's the main event, the heart attack. We believe that inflamed plaque is more dangerous than noninflamed plaque.

This is a Holy Grail of cardiology. How to sort out which plaque is vulnerable to rupture and which isn't.

———

The policeman today would have initiated CPR. Cardiac massage, at least. And you would call for the EMS, and they would have come and they would have shocked him.

That might have bought you enough time to transport him. But that is the difference between 1969 and now. In 1969, you did what you could.

As soon as your dad had his initial symptoms, his clock started. Today, from that moment to definite treatment is so much shorter than it was when he had his attack. Really, since [about] 1970 the whole push has been to get patients early, identify them early, be very aggressive. Extend the treatment out there into the community, and speed it up.

That was the whole idea of nine-one-one.

The paramedics would have arrived and determined that he was in ventricular disintegration. They would have done CPR, shocked him instantly, put an IV into him, and continued CPR while they transported him.

EMTs take EKGs right at the scene. They can transmit it to the ER, [where] the ER docs will tell [the EMTs] how to treat it. That's the lesson of your dad—that compared with what happened [to him], the care is so much closer to the people now. The extension of the care out to the community—instead of you running up and down the block to find a phone to call your mother.

Here in the emergency room, from the time a person hits the door until he gets a clot buster has to be no more than thirty minutes. Door-to-drug time. Door to cath lab—

with the needle in the groin—no more than ninety min-
utes. Every minute, the heart is dying.

If you had been fully trained [or] been an EMT, it [still]
would have done no good. . . . I can tell you with absolute
certainty, there was nothing you could have done for your
dad. . . . The chances would be maybe 50-50 today. . . .
Short of taking out your Boy Scout knife and slicing him
open and doing massage, there was nothing you could
have done. . . . It was nobody's fault. . . .

========

You say you felt a faint pulse. But at that point either way
it would have been completely ineffective.

In a heart attack, the event itself is sort of a continuum.
What happens—though we didn't know this back then—
is that the artery closes and the blood supply is cut off
from a section of the heart. When that happens, that part
of the heart muscle dies. What makes it lethal is that it ex-
poses the heart, that part of the heart, to electrical insta-
bility. This electrical instability creates ventricular
fibrillation, which causes sudden cardiac death. That's
what I think you [felt] that night.

Ventricular fibrillation is a very fine rapid movement, a
turbulence where nothing is really happening. . . .
Tachycardia is an organized heartbeat, but it is so fast
the heart can not fill [with blood]. It can be difficult to

tell if it's ventricular fibrillation or tachycardia. The heart has to fill before it can empty. If it gets going [too] fast there is not time to fill, and then it contracts while it's still empty.

When you run out of gas, you're done. When the ventricle loses its gas, it's done. Trickle, trickle, trickle down the highway, but [by then] it all just depends on how fast you were going.

[T]here are pacemaker cells in the upper part of the heart, called the atrium, that go down into the middle of the heart and down into the ventricles, which do the pumping. When atrial pacemaking function fails, you go into backup mode and the [pacemaker cells in the] middle tr[y] to take over the pacemaker function. When that fails it goes to another backup mode, and the lower part of the heart, the ventricular part, tries to take over. . . . When the heart can't do any of that, the pacemakers just go CRAZY. You don't have any pumping at all. You have a quivering heart, like a bowl of Jell-O.

I think of it as a bunch of kindergarten kids going absolutely crazy.

His heart was like a bag of worms. It's trying to work, but it's not. . . . A thousand worms moving around rapidly and very excitedly inside a little sack. . . . It doesn't have the strength or the correct electrical impulses to do its job. It's starving for air, twitching uncontrollably.

That's why perhaps you were able to feel a weak, rapid pulse of some sort. You could have been experiencing that there was still some fibrillation. But a lot of his heart was already dead.

[It] may have been the final run of ventricular tachycardia before the heart went into fibrillation and stopped for the final time.

His heart may have been intermittently kicking back into a normal rhythm. But it wasn't sustainable.

It's even money that the pulse you think you were feeling was your own. That's what happened when you tried to find it. The wrist is a terrible place to try to pick it up. What the policeman was doing, he was looking for the pulse on a carotid artery on his neck. That's harder to find, but it is definitely there.

Quite possibly what you felt were indeed his last few heartbeats, as his heart . . . just petered out.

———

From the hospital we repaired to Schmitts. Mom sat on the sofa by the far wall; I sat on the piano bench opposite, near the front door. Mr. Schmitt returned to the dining room table and started a list of who needed to be notified. Every so often he'd look up and ask Mom a question, usually for the name of a Cole Steel someone.

More York Crowd moms appeared. Mrs. Kirk. Mrs. Philbin. Mrs. Masterson. Word was traveling quickly. From my seat on the piano I served as doorman. When Mrs. Philbin came in I laughed a little, because I always laughed a little when I saw Mrs. Philbin. When I was serving Mass, if I saw Mrs. Philbin coming to the Communion rail, I had to avoid eye contact, because she could always make me laugh, and to giggle on the altar was the Unforgivable Sin. She knew it too, and she would always try to make me laugh even as I could see her fighting the very impulse. I opened the door and there she was and I laughed. For maybe the only time ever, she didn't.

Then Mrs. Masterson came in. She hurried past me, wound her way urgently between the chairs and the coffee table, and wedged herself down on the sofa between Mom and the mom next to her. She draped her right arm around Mom, leaned into her, and with that commenced to weep uncontrollably, huge wails, unashamed and unembarrassed. I had never seen anything like it before in my life. It was stunning in its nakedness. She was completely unafraid—of herself or her emotions, and until she had wrung herself out, Mom and the rest of us in Schmitt's living room were at a standstill.

The Mastersons were one of the last of the York Crowd families to get to Haines Acres. They had moved from Chicago into their house on Eastwood Drive in July 1964, earlier by one month than we had moved from Wilshire Drive to Stanford. Sitting at Schmitts, I remembered the first time she had come over to our house, the two moms reaching out to each other in the time-honored, St. Joe's way. She and Mom had met through the women's bowling league. Now five years later here she wept, making for me the unreal very real.

That once more the York Crowd moms were drawing together, this time here at Schmitts, was both appropriate and no accident. Years later, but well before any notion that I would write this book, Mr. Leahy and I were having a conversation about the York Crowd and its dynamic. Mr. and Mrs. Leahy were another of the last families to get to York and St. Joe's. He observed that whatever it was that had worked so well, the credit belonged exclusively to the moms. Roles were clearly defined then. Some would say "rigidly." And the economics were such for these middle-class dads that many of the moms did not have to work (outside the home), and most chose not to. Mom was one of the few who did, actually, much to Dad's chagrin, I think. He was the "breadwinner," back before that word was fraught with connotation. But Mr. Leahy was correct about the York Crowd. It was the moms who created it, nurtured it, sustained it. Without the moms, there could be no crowd. The dads' job was to go off in the morning to their high-powered careers and then come back home at 6:00 P.M. The moms? They did everything else.

At one point at Schmitts, apropos of nothing (because everything was now apropos of nothing), Mom said that a priest from St. Joe's had been at the hospital to give Dad Last Rites. "He said Dad was in good shape," Mom announced, and it was good to hear. Interesting, too, that it would have been this priest, given the moment here at Schmitts. He was a firebrand, eager to mix it up from the pulpit. His directive (every Sunday, it seemed): Husbands, respect your wives. He didn't preach, he harangued. I didn't pay him much mind. He wasn't talking to me, and he sure wasn't funny. Only now, in retrospect, do I find him fascinating.

If the dads were the chairmen of their family corporations, coming and going as needed, the moms were the chief executive officers, forever on the job. Noreen has said that the larger world missed out on many talented people back then, all of those women who could have been running the store if only they'd been given the opportunity—or, perhaps, thought to want to. They were purchasing agents, office managers, scheduling secretaries, senior accountants, general traffic managers, efficiency experts, quality-and-assurance executives. Speaking in general terms here, I don't believe their husbands took them for granted. It is worth noting that among these York Crowd couples—all told with the comings and goings, the number over the years grew to probably twenty-five—there was not a single divorce among them. But I also believe that a husband's job description in those days did not include being aware of what all their wives were up to when they were off at work cranking the postwar engine. Again, in retrospect only do I understand that there was a complex, delicately balanced dance taking place between these men and women, these husbands and wives, these moms and dads. But for better and worse, the 1950s and 1960s couldn't have happened without this arrangement, and we will likely never see its like again. I don't doubt this could be confining for the moms. But in its way, I think, it also had to be freeing. These women were *in charge*. They most certainly were at Schmitts that night. And if the business world didn't benefit from their myriad skills, all of us kids surely did.

These moms were the event planners and communication specialists of their day, long before the words were invented. They gathered regularly. (And still do: there remains an afternoon bridge club that can trace its lineage back nearly fifty years.) These moms ruled. For a couple of autumns when I was in grade school, some of the families headed three hours north for a weekend at the cabins at Worlds End State Park near Forksville, Pennsylvania, birthplace of Red Grange, football's Galloping Ghost. It was a terrific time, everyone returning home Sunday night reeking of smoke and spaghetti sauce. The first year it was an exhilarating dash thrown together at the last minute. This idea, I'd wager, came from the moms, who told the dads, and away we went.

Sometimes the dads would take the sons on an overnight tent-camping trip to Caledonia State Park, west of Gettysburg, with Dad serving as guide. Even that was probably the moms' idea. *You're going*. We had spur-of-the-moment trips to the Stony Brook Drive-In Theater, all us kids in our pajamas, where we parked the cars in every other stall and put the lawn chairs in between. There was the caravan to Painters Mill Music Fair, a summer-stock theater in Owings Mills, Maryland. The excursion in 1962 remains special to me, if no one else. We saw Darren McGavin as Harold Hill in *The Music Man*. I was nine years old, and I followed his career until he died in 2006. Whether he was Carl Kolchak on *The Night Stalker*, the uncredited Gus Sands in *The Natural*, or Candice Bergen's father on *Murphy Brown*, he was to me always the "Ol' Perfesser," charming Marian Paroo in the River City, Iowa, library.

If you grew up a baby-boom kid, you had Depression-era parents. Ergo, you learned the value of a dollar, through lessons like this one, taught by the moms. The second Tuesday of September was the opening day of the York Fair, a countywide extravaganza. The schools let out at noon to get as many kids as possible through the turnstiles. Nothing doing, said our moms, at least back before any of us were in high school. We went on a picnic to Samuel S. Lewis State Park, southeast of York. They sold it to us with the promise that we'd have the place to ourselves, which proved true. It was a great spot, atop Mount Pisgah with its view of the Susquehanna River valley. There were rocks to climb and trees to scale, and there was always an acorn fight, boys against the girls. You could tell which of the older boys liked which of the older girls because they would be throwing the most acorns at each other. When we got home Kathy and I would wait for Dad so we could tell him all about it, about everything that he had missed because he had to be at work. It would be years before I recognized the money-saving scam the moms had perpetrated.

Mrs. Philbin, Mrs. Flick, and Mom started the girls' basketball program at St. Joe's, though only Mrs. Philbin had ever played the game. This was in the very early 1960s, when women's athletics were ignored at best, an unspeakable act at worst. The game was six on six, with the girls playing either defense or offense but not both, with no running past half-court. The contests themselves were a maddening series of clock-stopping jump balls. But it was a beginning, and they persevered. Kathy can still go into paroxysms of laughter when talking of an uninhibited Mrs. Philbin demonstrating how to establish a pivot foot and then *reeeeaaaching* with her other leg—in unfettered, fully unladylike fashion—to gain position. The girls went wide-eyed with horror, utterly appalled at the very idea. Mrs. Philbin went on to coach the York Catholic basketball team for a year or two when these St. Joe's girls got a bit older. Again, a beginning. In 1979, the days of Mrs. Philbin and the rest by then forgotten, the York Catholic girls won a state championship.

But for all that can be remembered of the big events, the important moments, as with all things York Crowd, the moms' real value was cemented in the small stuff, in the day-to-day that must get done and is then dismissed. This list has no end. Here is one item to represent them all, suggested by Mrs. McEntee. In the early days, when Haines Acres was just a few blocks without sewers or sidewalks and St. Joe's elementary was downtown, there was no bus service to get the kids back and forth. "We had to call each other and figure it out," Mrs. McEntee said. Who would drive in and who would pick up, on what days. To complicate logistics, there weren't many two-car families. And often as not, the phone call would be the first time the two moms had spoken to each other. It was the moms who made the York Crowd happen, from day one.

I sometimes think I have spent the rest of my life trying to duplicate what those women created for me, that protective and protected sense of community, and not just on the night Dad died. I have had some success with this, as Mom herself noted up in Fairbanks. Noreen and I also have another group of close friends with whom we have shared much of the last twenty-five years. It began when we moved to Brooklyn in 1982 and were introduced to them through my cousin Peter Callaghan, Aunt Marg's son, and his partner, West. We are scattered now across New Hampshire, Albany and Troy, New York, and Brooklyn, but long ago we consciously began organizing our next outing while the current one was under way. The Christmas party is at our house. The winter bonfire on a New Hampshire farm is a huge conflagration that has grown to primal significance, the orange sparks rising to the white dots in a black sky. Five children have now been gathered round. It is a good night.

Also, Noreen and I joined the Oratory Church of St. Boniface in downtown Brooklyn. We found the place when the St. Joe's church building in downtown York was desanctified, a new one built out in . . . Haines Acres. St. Joe's had remained "my" church, even though I showed up there only two or three times a year. The new building is beautiful, I'm sure, but it will never be St. Joe's for me. Suddenly churchless, St. Boniface filled the void—a relatively new parish in an old church structure, not unlike Mom and Dad's situation new to York in the 1950s. I believe I am like Dad when it comes to my Catholicism. I am by no means spiritual, nor am I particularly religious. But I value the community—the primacy of the people, the importance of the gathered. A few years ago a St. Boniface parishioner collapsed and died while out for a run. He was in his late forties. His wake was at Bonnie's. I had known him only to say hello, but I had to attend. The viewing was packed, like at Dad's. I understood and felt at home. No, I was home. More recently, I realized I was attending church on Sundays to see who else was there, to say hello to new acquaintances becoming old friends. St. Joe's repeating itself.

When I was a junior in high school, living at York Catholic, rehearsing *Brigadoon*, I asked Mom if I could have Mr. Leahy come to a rehearsal to help the kids with the Scottish burr. He was great with accents. Mom said no. But, she said, I could ask him to go to a rehearsal and then with the rest of his family come to our house for dinner. After all, he would be giving up a Sunday afternoon. Years later, when Patrick was in fourth grade, I organized an ice-skating club at his school, a Fridays-through-the-winter thing. I pulled out all the stops. A weekly newsletter, for instance, typed, copied, stamped, and mailed in that final mid-1990s moment before e-mail overwhelmed us. I put all the kids in garish yellow stocking caps that I had purchased from a street vendor, and we called ourselves the Golden Hawks Skate Club. Though the real purpose for the hats was so I could keep track of them at the Prospect Park rink. Nothing like this had been done before at the school. The parents were very appreciative and they said so, with a few presenting me with cases of beer, or bottles of Baileys Irish Cream. But only one couple took it to the next level, the York level. The mom joined the club for a Friday skate, and then Noreen and Patrick and I went to their place for homemade chili. Sitting at their table, I felt an old familiarity. The attention to detail. Of the twelve sets of parents from the skate club, this is the one with whom we have become real friends.

———

Mom made one other out-of-nowhere comment at Schmitts that night, before the two of us went up to Philbins. Another non sequitur, apropos of nothing. "Well," she said, "at least I wasn't mad at him." I have always taken this declaration at face value—even now, when I know that for Mom and Dad, separately and together, the last few years contained their struggles. Mom's comment eased the tension a bit, just a bit, and from around the living room there came from the gathered moms a few commiserating chuckles, knowing shakes of the head, arching eyebrows of shared experience. There would always be much to learn from these women.

TUESDAY,
SEPTEMBER 30, 10:20 P.M.

I WAS TAKING HIS PULSE WHEN IT STOPPED. THAT'S HOW I REMEM-
ber it. There was a new show on TV, *Marcus Welby, M.D.* Dad
had just come downstairs from the kitchen, with another Coke
or maybe a beer, and I told him what was going on. Robert
Young from the old *Father Knows Best* was a family doctor
who was getting a little older. He'd had a mild heart attack, so
he'd brought in this new young wet-fish doctor to work with
him. We took our assigned seats. Dad in his chair, the left side
of the sofa; me in the upholstered rocker, the one I really liked
because I could throw my right leg over the arm, sit kind of
sideways and swing back and forth and spin around a little,
too. Then it happened, and not many minutes later I was taking his pulse when it stopped.

Dad was in a great mood that night. I mean terrific. Laughing,
joking. Ask Mom and she'll say the same thing. It's about all
she says about that night.

Dinner was fun. If there was any Cole Steel dramaturgy, it
was dispensed with quickly. In truth, dinner usually was a

pleasant time—once we got past Dad's story of the day and except on those nights when I brought my report card home from school and Mom said, *Your father gets to enjoy his dinner before seeing that.* Fridays were especially fun. For Kathy and me because there was no school the next day, for Dad maybe because there was some hunting or fishing in store, or even if he was going to work he'd be in flannel shirt and paint-spattered khakis with the pocket full of change to buy his forklift guys and truck drivers cups of lousy coffee. There was also spaghetti and clam sauce on the table. Helen O'Neil from Irish Buffalo learned to cook Italian when she moved to Pennsylvania Dutch Country. Yo Rudnick taught her. She was Italian, married to the Jewish Leo Rudnick, a Cole Steel colleague of Dad's. York had become something of a melting pot after all. Mom still laughs when recalling Mrs. Rudnick's universal direction: "First, sauté some garlic in olive oil." And Friday night was often coin night. After dinner Dad would spill the contents of his pocket on the table, maybe augment it with the change he'd been dropping on his night stand during the week, and we'd go through it looking for dates to press into the empty circles in our blue-cardboard coin-collecting folders. A 1909 Lincoln Head penny was one of his great finds, though I always liked the 1943 steel pennies he came home with now and again.

On this night, Dad regaled us with the story of his drive home from work, having great fun poking fun at himself. He'd gotten one of those pains in his back, the ones that made him arch his back crazily and throw his arms back if he was going to get it to go away. Except now he was on Route 83 where there

was a series of overpasses above the Codorus Creek and an industrial section near Cole Steel. The pavement sections were
kind of dippy, one after the other, and at the right speed the
car would undulate in this weird roly-poly rhythm. You're going to know how only if you drive it every day. So here he was
hitting it at just the right MPH when the pains hit him, and
he's got his back arched and head back and his arms yanked
behind him as far as he can and still hold the wheel. Now
here's where it got real funny for Dad, telling the story and
laughing. He's slowing down now because he can barely grip
the wheel, and so cars start passing on the left. And Dad just
knew everybody was turning to look at him. He's wearing his
hat—he forgot to say he was wearing his hat!—and the brim
was rolled up all the way around, so he must have looked like
Frank Fontaine's Crazy Guggenheim talking to Jackie Glea-
son's Joe the Bartender, all bug eyes, weird grin, and goofy
topper.

There was more laughter that night. Dad did have a terrific
sense of humor, a crafty way about him. Among the York
Crowd, he and Mrs. Schmitt sported a well-deserved (some
probably said notorious) reputation as table-talkers when
paired in bridge. Something between them just clicked. Or as
Mrs. Bauler remarked, "I liked the way he would get this sly
little smile on his face. It was like he already knew the punch
line of the next joke." Dad once sat me down in front of the
TV to watch the comic Guy Marks perform his bird and insect
impersonation, with orders not to forget. Kathy says she can
still hear him down in the TV room, cackling at Rowan &
Martin, the famous 1960s comedy team. The pre-*Laugh-In*

Rowan & Martin on *The Dean Martin Show*. They had this routine in which they were trench-coated spies, and after backing into each other Dan Rowan would start in with a ridiculously complicated series of instructions to an increasingly befuddled Dick Martin, yet somehow Martin repeated the instructions word for word a mere millisecond behind Rowan. Dad always wondered if Rowan made up his instructions on the fly to try to trip up Martin, elevating the whole thing near to genius. But the funny part—wait, Dad would say, here comes the funny part!—was when Rowan suddenly stopped and asked, "Got that?" and one perfect beat later Martin delivered his iconic line: "I lost you at the bakery!" And Dad would howl.

He watched *Teacher's Pet* whenever it came on TV. Clark Gable, Doris Day, and especially Gig Young, who at one point is nursing a hilariously horrible hangover and when the doorbell rings he stumbles over and desperately grabs at the long chimes, begging for the noise to stop. On Sunday nights during the fall of 1968, Dad followed the campaign of the phlegmatic, stone-faced Pat Paulsen, running for president on *The Smothers Brothers Comedy Hour*. There were the albums of Elaine May and Mike Nichols, Bob Newhart, and, a little later, Bill Cosby, all spun on our gigantic hi-fi. The comics Jonathan Winters and Charlie Callas, the impersonators David Frye and Rich Little. I mention them all because at the kitchen table that night Dad, Mom, and I took turns mimicking one of his favorites, I just can't remember who. It might have been Red Skelton, maybe Dad's all-time all-timer. Skelton had been on *The Ed Sullivan Show* just that Sunday night past, and we might have seen him. Whatever. Whomever. Dinner was silly and it got sillier. I see Dad laughing, relaxed and happy.

"When the legend becomes fact, print the legend." So said the newspaper man in *The Man Who Shot Liberty Valance,* the classic John Ford western. Truth said John Wayne; myth said Jimmy Stewart. The *Shinbone Star* stuck with Stewart. Here is our legend: Dad was in a merry mood for more reasons than just his driving story or our dumb impersonations. In the drawer of his night stand upstairs lay a letter of resignation, dated October 1, 1969, that Dad planned to deliver to the office powers the next morning. Mom found it many months later when she could finally bring herself to clean out the drawer—filled, surely, with half-eaten rolls of Tums, stray salt pills, maybe five dollars in change, and probably some old rosary beads, expired hunting and fishing licenses, a couple of spent shotgun shells, fishing line, lots of pens and pencils, and who knows how many pieces of paper, maybe an old one from Mom to the South Pacific, perhaps a new one with a few tersely typed paragraphs folded into an envelope.

Kathy insists on this, saying she can see Mom as she's telling her, and I surely want to believe. Were this a novel, I wouldn't dare make it up. Nor this: "I know," says Mr. Ochs, the fishing buddy who helped Dad up the hill. "I *know* that your Dad carried a resignation letter in his pocket around with him at Cole Steel the last few years." It had become that kind of place. If word got out the hatchet man was on the prowl, maybe Dad could get his head off the chopping block in time. "That way your Dad would never get fired."

Mom, however, says she remembers nothing of a letter, in Dad's pocket or his night stand. But there is fact here, she says. I learned of it many years later. A few weekends before Tuesday, Dad had driven home from a job interview with a company in Maryland, picked up Mom, and together they went to dinner to celebrate. He was to be the top man of the traffic department, *running his own show*. Dad would commute for the rest of my senior year at York Catholic. After I went to college up at Niagara, they'd move but remain close enough to still be part of the York Crowd, if not on an everyday basis. The money was great—twenty thousand plus! It was all coming together, the hard work of a lifetime. And Dad would be done with Cole Steel.

Since Monday was my night to do the dishes, Mom likely cleaned up after dinner and then headed down to Schmitts. Perhaps I had some homework, but at 8:30 I was downstairs with Dad in the TV room. There was a new ABC Movie of the Week I wanted to watch that looked good. It was called *The Immortal.* A man discovers, after donating blood, that he is immune to all disease, and the billionaire who gets saved by a transfusion then tries to turn him into his own private blood bank. This guy is a test-car driver, and at the end he makes his escape in a green Mustang. Neat. I wanted to see it because it starred Christopher George, who a couple of years before had been in *The Rat Patrol,* a very cool World War II series about four soldiers running their jeeps up and down sand dunes while battling Rommel in North Africa. George wore an Australian hat, the brim on the left side pinned up jauntily. But one of the other soldiers wore what looked like a Civil War infantry hat with his goggles perched on top. To this day I like that look—sunglasses pushed out of the way over the brim of a baseball cap. In *The Immortal,* Dad was pleased to see Barry Sullivan, hollow cheeks and all, as the bad guy. Sullivan had been in one of Dad's favorite TV westerns, *The Tall Man,* as the sheriff Pat Garrett.

Dad's all-time TV Western, though, was probably *Have Gun—Will Travel,* with Richard Boone as Paladin. He was by turns a Shakespeare-quoting, card-playing San Francisco swell or a black-clad bounty hunter with a white knight insignia on his holster and a highly developed, quirky sense of right and wrong. I have glommed that description from various Internet sites, but I remember clearly the appeal this character held for Dad.

My favorite western, and Kathy's, too, had been *The Adventures of Rin Tin Tin.* Though we rarely saw it. It aired in the late 1950s and was on ABC, and our TV barely pulled in the required Philadelphia station. But we'd try, and sometimes we'd get a snowy image. If we were lucky it would be an episode that featured Tom McKee, our Uncle Tom McKee, Dad's older brother. He played Captain Davis.

Uncle Tom and Dad had shared the unheated trek up the back stairs to the attic bedroom on Rodney Avenue when they were boys. Dad didn't talk much about him, and I don't think they had much contact with each other. Though Dad spoke quite fondly of a couple of boyhood summers when he and Tom, the city boys, were literally farmed out to a working spread in Ohio where the two brothers side by side milked the cows and mucked the stalls. Dad remembered this with enough fondness that once while on a vacation out that way we went looking for the place, though we never found it.

Tom moved to Los Angeles after the war and amassed a lengthy, workmanlike string of credits in TV shows and movies. A line here, a spot there, often playing the unshaven tough-guy ranch hand or platoon-member leatherneck. Throw in the commercial work and radio voice-overs that Uncle Tom likely did to pay the bills for a wife and kids, and he had the kind of successful career any struggling actor would kill for.

Once, home from college in the early 1970s, I was off to bed when *The Court-Martial of Billy Mitchell* came on the *Late Show*. It starred Gary Cooper as the Army Air Corps flier famously put on trial in 1925 for questioning his superiors. "Uncle Tom's in this," Mom said. So of course we stayed up. Since Mom couldn't remember when he might appear on screen—or for how long—we watched intently, never blinking. Indeed, while we waited, Darren McGavin appeared as a pilot forever loyal to Mitchell. And then suddenly there was Uncle Tom. Seeing his face took my breath away, jolted me, snapped me to attention. He was playing Eddie Rickenbacker, in a spirited thirty-second exchange with Ralph Bellamy, but he was Dad. There was the same full, rich hair, swept back on either side, the severe widow's peak, the intense brow. And of course the "McKee Nose," too big for the rest of him. He looked just like Dad, especially through the lips (thin) and jaw (square). Mom said that in real life Uncle Tom's hair was darker, but the movie color lent everything a reddish cast, making him all the more

Dad. It was perfectly stunning. My father alive again, here in our TV room.

The Immortal done, Dad and I moved right into *Marcus Welby, M.D.* A brand new series in just its second show, it had been last week's number one and was on the cover of *TV GUIDE*. Dad went up to the kitchen, and when he came back I filled him in: some parents had a kid with mental problems, and they didn't know what to do.

I heard it before I saw it. The sound of air being pulled through tightly clenched teeth. By the time I turned to look at him, I'd heard it twice. Dad's eyes were wide open, his brows pushed up onto his forehead, his lips pulled wide across his mouth in a leering, maniacal grin. He looked like the pictures I'd seen of the astronauts' faces on the rocket sled, their faces yanked back by the G-force. With every gasp his back slammed into the couch and stayed there, stuck to it, as if there were someone or something behind the couch holding on to him. Then suddenly the gasp would stop, and for a split second time stood still, until the hand behind the couch pushed him forward violently, only to grab him and pull him right back when the gasping started again. And there would be this thumping noise, like a fist was hitting him in the chest. He was so straight and stiff against the sofa it was like he had a metal rod jammed down his spine, right through his head.

By now I was standing over him. I had leapt up before the third gasp. I yelled at him—"Dad! Dad! Dad!"—but he was hearing nothing. I wanted to put a hand on his shoulder, to keep him from lunging again, but I was afraid to touch him. In the moment between the gasp and the next pitch forward and all the thumping I could see right into his eyes, but there was nothing there. No life. No terror. Nothing.

I ran up the stairs to the kitchen, to the phone. Nine-one-one? York wouldn't have the emergency number for another nine months. Mom, I had to get to Mom. I picked up the receiver, on the kitchen wall by the dining room. Nothing. No dial tone, anything. Dead as Dad. In a burst I thought this through. This wasn't unusual, for one thing. Or at least it happened enough to know the cause and not to worry. Haines Acres was in another building boom, and it seemed like every other week some construction crew was cutting another phone line. Service would be back in a couple of hours. I yelled at the receiver, slammed it down, and bounded down the steps into the TV room.

Dad was still doing the same thing, only now there was spit and mucous and this puffy, white stuff oozing from the corner of his mouth onto his shirt—more coming out with every sharp, gaggy breath. With the phone out, I needed help. I sprinted outside and then came to a stop on the front porch. What do I do? I decided to head up the hill to our next-door neighbors. There were lights on and I banged on the door a couple of times, but nothing. I took off down the hill, past our house—I'd left the front door open and you could see the glow of the TV from the sidewalk—to our neighbors on the other side. It was amazing we were still friends. A couple of years ago the husband had appeared at our house holding a twig. Actually it wasn't a twig, it was some sort of exotic Asian tree that he had recently planted and that our mutt Kelly had even more recently chewed off right at the dirt. We had not only remained friends, the wife then proceeded to fall in love with our dog, who now stayed with her during the day eating ice cream and all other manner of things, lugging himself up the hill only when I got home from school.

I ran past the long row of hyacinth that separated our houses. Their place was dark and looked deserted. I sprinted across the lawn and up the front steps and rang the bell and pounded on the door. I rang again and pounded again, then screamed at them for good measure and took off, back up the hill and into our house.

Everything was different now. No back and forth. Nothing. A different nothing. Dad had slid forward on the sofa, barely still sitting at all, just his arms twitching, his knees jutting out into the living room way past his feet, which were tucked up underneath him. He was leaning a bit to his right, his chin flat on his chest, his mouth flopped open, the white stuff he had been spewing before when gasping now oozing onto his shirt in gobs. I bent down and looked at him. I called his name. "Dad! Dad!" I ran upstairs into Mom and Dad's bedroom to get a blanket, came down, and wrapped it around him, taking care to cover him completely and tuck it around his chin. Then I stood up, alone in the room.

I have said before that Dad rarely talked to me about his own father. The one time he did proves this rule. A Saturday morning in February 1968. I know the particulars because we were in the coffee shop of a Holiday Inn–like place somewhere near

Shamokin. The night before some of the York Crowd families—McKees, Philbins, Gradys, and Byrnes, as I recall—had
made another of their trips, this time to watch York Catholic
play Our Lady of Lourdes in basketball, and then we all stayed
overnight.

The next morning it was just Dad and me together at
breakfast. And from out of nowhere—completely out of
nowhere—Dad started talking about his father. Maybe because we were up in Pennsylvania coal country, up near
where Jack McKee had lived as a kid that had triggered an
old-time remembrance. Though it soon became something
else altogether different.

Jack McKee was fifteen when his father died—of a heart attack, of course—leaving him more or less on his own. He lived
in Scranton, Pennsylvania. To support himself, he found work
as a plasterer, going where the work was, even as young as he
was, from Scranton west to Erie, Pennsylvania, and up into
western New York and over to eastern Ohio and sometimes
farther. That's how he and Nana had met. Anna Carey worked
at a boarding house where Jack bunked. Of all the boarding
houses in Buffalo. . . . There were lots of them, then, with
most of the men working the granaries. This one was barely
around the corner from where Nana lived. Dad pointed to the
plaster ceiling. His dad always used to sign his work, Dad said,
the way all plasterers did. There was probably a signature up
there somewhere. What they would do was find an out-of-the-
way spot and while the plaster was still a bit wet etch their
name into it, then let it set some more. Before it was completely dry, they'd come back with a trowel and fill in the name

with a bit of newer, wetter plaster and smooth it over. Because of the different drying times between the two layers, the scratched-in *Jack McKee* would disappear to the eye but be there all the same.

Great stuff. All of it. My grandfather alive to me on the strength of his signature. However, when the legend becomes fact. . . .

My great-grandfather Frank McKee died on November 26, 1913, "at his home . . . after a lingering illness," according to the *Scranton Times*. "Apoplexy," says the death certificate, with the doctor of record attending for six months. It was probably a stroke, still in keeping with the McKees' cardiovascular conundrum. He was fifty-three years old. He had for years worked as a brakeman, flagman, watchman, switch tender, and old-fashioned laborer, mostly for the Delaware Lackawanna & Western Railroad. He was born in Philadelphia and was married to the former Mary Ann Cannon of Scranton. They had eight surviving children. My grandfather was the second oldest and the oldest of the four boys. Age matters here. In 1913, Jack McKee was twenty-five years old, not fifteen. He wasn't exactly on his own, either, what with all those brothers and sisters.

The rest of Dad's story is pretty much fact. Jack McKee had worked for a couple of years as a "driver," a "fireman," and as a plain "laborer," according to Scranton city directories. These were probably mining jobs; there were plenty of them, and the Cayuga shaft was within walking distance of Oak Street. He did take off on his own after his father died, and it isn't hard to figure why. He was still living at home, sleeping upstairs with all those brothers and sisters in a four-room, two-story house that was maybe twenty-by-fifteen feet, the second floor little more than an attic. Somewhere between Scranton and Buffalo he took up plastering. He met Nana, likely at a boarding house on Buffalo's Lower West Side where he was living and she was working. And he still occasionally went where the jobs took him. Aunt Alice has a letter he wrote to her from Lexington, Kentucky, in May 1941, two months before he would have his heart attack. He had found work around the Kentucky Derby, a good situation for a guy who followed the horses. Whirlaway by eight lengths, Eddie Arcaro up, on their way to a Triple Crown. Jack McKee wasn't a betting man, but maybe he won himself a couple of bucks anyway.

Did Dad have this story wrong and make a mistake? Or did he tell it wrong on purpose? I think the latter. I think he knew the facts but wanted some legend, and it was better served by a boy at fifteen than a man at twenty-five. There was a weirdness to our entire conversation at that breakfast, everything about it a half-beat off. Maybe because we were even *having* the conversation, my dad talking about his dad. But there was something else about it, and I sensed it even in the moment, making it all doubly weird. Dad was telling me something much more profound than just the saga of his father on his own, making his way. That was compelling enough. No, this was Dad's valedictory, his goodbye speech . . . to me. That's why it was so unsettling. I got it. I understood. Dad was saying goodbye to me. I am more convinced of it now. Can you imagine, Steve? Dad asked, and he kept asking.

What would you do, Steve, what would you do if you were on your own?

So panic feels like this, does it. A statement, not a question. Standing in the TV room, with no idea what to do next, it had me surrounded. I'd tried the phone. I'd gotten a blanket. I'd run to the neighbors. That was all I could do? Despair crept at me. I had to get help. I ran out of the house again—jumping the bushes in front of the porch—up the hill to our neighbors beyond the ones next door. I didn't even know who they were. I was well past the first house, sprinting hard for the next, when a Springettsbury Township Police car popped over the hill, cruising down Stanford Drive. This was most unusual. Except for those times when a construction crew had cut the phone lines. I turned on a dime and took off after him, right into the street, giving chase. I screamed but he didn't hear. The car kept moving, though slowly enough that I was actually overtaking it. I leaned in—one final sprint to the finishing tape, Tommie Smith, John Carlos, and me. Finally I got close enough to pound on the trunk with both fists. That brought the cruiser to an immediate halt right in front of our house. Momentum slammed me into the bumper and sprawled me over the trunk, which got the policeman out of his car in a hurry.

For the first time, I told my story. The cop then walked into our house. Of all the things I remember best of this night, that the cop *walked* into our house remains to this day at the top of the list. Inside, Dad was unchanged, his arms now still and lifeless, eerily suspended between toppling over and staying upright, still wrapped completely in the green blanket, a smear of white mucous coating the right side. The cop reached for his radio with his left hand, and with his right he pulled off the blanket and threw it on the floor. Dad didn't move, still slumped to the right, the sofa cushion beneath him now gone a darker brown around him. I sat down next to him, and from that angle it was impossible not to look right into his eyes, the green crystals that had seen me so proudly after *Brigadoon*, so angrily the night we had almost come to blows right here in this TV room. I would have taken either one of those looks now, either one, but he stared past me.

The cop hooked his right index finger under Dad's chin and flipped his head back, searching. That put Dad's face directly under the lamp on the side table. His mouth was agape, his hair askew, so unlike him, his skin a chalky gray, as if someone had erased a blackboard but really only pushed a dusting across the surface. The dark stubble of his five o'clock shadow stood out against it. Dad would want to get that shaved off first thing tomorrow morning. Finding a pulse seemed a good idea. I took hold of Dad's right hand and put my fingers on his wrist, searching for . . . what? Then I found it. I could feel it, at least I told the cop I could. Slow beats. Not much, but it was there. Then it took off like a machine gun for a long second, shot a few weak ones, then nothing. I told the cop he was dead. I looked again at Dad, watched as his head slowly rolled to the right, facing me. His right eye was closed now; the left stared straight ahead. He wasn't Dad. I couldn't see him, not anymore. I dropped his wrist and ran out the door, down the hill, into the night.

EPILOGUE

After all that and I nearly missed the start. Actually I did miss it. I was back in the holding area eating another banana, checking my bike one more time, making sure my helmet was balanced just so on the handlebars for a quick grab during the transition. Or doing something to quell the nerves. I had just spent two months training for this triathlon and now the gun had gone off and I'd been caught standing. In fact, I don't think I officially entered the race because of it. By the time I ran from the holding area to the course, the main pack was up the road. I took a short-cut to catch up, so the computer chip on my ankle bracelet never crossed the electronic starting line.

Once on the course I tried to settle into my snail's-pace jog. I checked my heart monitor, though I didn't have to. I could tell I had already blown past my 80 percent maximum of 133 beats per minute. I knew it. I glanced at the wristwatch dial: "141." One hundred forty-one, and I was maybe one minute into a race that figured to take me a solid hour and forty-five minutes on a good day. I was also at some altitude, probably about 4,400 feet. Not a lot, but enough. Dr. Fein at the Princeton Longevity Center had been very enthusiastic that I try this tri. "No reason not to," he said. "You're in great shape." I may have failed to mention the altitude part. I would have to slow down, at least for a while, bringing my jog to something very much like a walk. I had to be smart. Had to. Though meanwhile up ahead there was Patrick, running backward, a big grin on his face, his hands spinning the international sign for "Hurry UP, Dad. *Cummmm-aaawn!*"

It fell on me from out of the sky, this triathlon. It was meant to be. That's how I saw it. When I left the Princeton Longevity Center I was worried that I would never set foot inside a gym again, never get on the rowing machine, lift the weights, anything. What was the point? I had failed. I was utterly devastated, unable even to articulate what it was that had left me in shambles. It wasn't just the fact that I had heart disease. In its own weird way, that might not have been it at all. No, driving silently back to Brooklyn, Noreen sitting next to me, what stung was (the way I saw it) the fact that I had become that part of Dad I had worked so hard never to be. Because if I had heart disease, then wasn't I just like him? The Dad I had come to know in those six years between his heart attacks. The sullen Dad, the depressed Dad. The Dad who gave up; the Dad who wasn't quite alive. That isn't all of who he was in those six years—I have a need to stress that—but it had become the part of him that I had come to know the best. And I didn't like him, that bit of him. Driving back to Brooklyn I felt like I was going to jump right out of my skin, the way Kathy said Dad must have felt whenever he tried to give up smoking.

It was Noreen who dragged me through that first weekend, mainly by saying almost nothing. When she did talk, it was next to nothing. "You're still here, Steve," she said. To her it was that plain, that straightforward. "You're still here."

Dr. Fein had said as much during our consult. "There is basically no end to the ways that having kept yourself fit has improved your situation," he said. I'd lowered my insulin levels, improved my blood lipids, built collateral arteries in my heart around any blockages, to name just a few. The list, he said, was endless. I would probably already have had a heart attack by now—at best. More likely, I probably wouldn't be alive to be getting this news. I was even paying forward, banking reserves on any heart attack that I might someday have. "The odds that you'll do well if you ever do have a heart attack are very high," he said, the most left-handed compliment I have ever heard.

He talked of death. "It can be difficult to accept one's mortality," he said. But I didn't think then, and I don't think now, that this was about death. I faced my mortality on September 30, 1969. The night I watched Dad die I watched me die, too. My life began the night his ended. *Learn from me*, he said. And so I did. I have become who I am because of him, because of that night. I can't imagine my life without all that running and rowing and biking and all the rest. Every other day after day. It's who I am, because of him. And I am alive.

Not that I knew this driving home from the PLC. My worry then was that I would bag it all, forget it. What was the point? It hadn't worked. That was on Friday. But by the following Thursday I was back in the gym. Because where else was I to go? I punished the rowing machine, punished me, rowing myself to near exhaustion. A thirty-two-minute, 7,000-meter pull. I did it because. Because I could. It left me slumped in my seat, chest heaving, my heart and I screaming at each other.

Yes! This is what I could do, because I always have: exercise. So I decided to do something . . . official. A row, a run, something that would require its own dedication, specific planning. Another Equinox of some sort. As to what, I hadn't a clue. And then this triathlon fell on me from the sky. Patrick was enrolled in a new school where the disciplines of the swim-bike-run were part of the program. The first weekend in November would be the classic "Turkey Tri," with parents invited to help with registration, to hand out water, to keep order at the finish line. Or if they wanted, we were told, they were certainly welcome to participate. Thank you. Thank you very much.

———

On October 10, 2005, a 2,000-word version of my trip to the PLC appeared in a *Wall Street Journal Report*. My lifelong promise keeping; the unexpected diagnosis; the recommendation of a cholesterol-lowering statin drug; my (very, very) begrudging acquiescence.

That was a Monday. My day on the Global Copy Desk begins at 3:30 P.M. There were perhaps fifty e-mails waiting for me when I arrived at my desk. By the end of the week there were more than a hundred. I would receive 226 total. The last one arrived nearly four months after the article appeared. *I was throwing out some old newspapers when I came across . . .*

These e-mails ran the full spectrum of emotions, points of view, suggestions, beliefs. By some I was roundly criticized.

Your sources are flawed. Most doctors and scientists, and the government in particular, are influenced by the dairy industry, the meat industry, and the pharmaceutical industry. And on and on [to the special-interest] lobbies who only care about the bottom line rather than the public's health.

Your article is a paid political commercial for the drug companies.

What is the take-home message . . . ? . . . "[H]ey, look at me . . . If I can get [coronary artery disease] with my lifestyle, you poor fat lazy bastards are all out of luck."

Stay away from the fear mongers who are selling snake oil.

Others used the moment as a bully pulpit to vent their view that the medical establishment and the insurance industry put the emphasis on the back end of treatment and not the front end of prevention. Too many people have coronary heart disease and don't know it, wrote one doctor, and "their first symptom is their last (sudden cardiac death). It is an amazing fact. Coronary artery disease is the #1 killer in this country and yet as a medical profession we are not aggressive in making diagnosis early."

Seventeen people recommended twenty-two books. Lifestyle tomes. Diet plans. Self-help manuals. Two authors sent me their books. Seventeen doctors of various stripe offered second opinions. Most of them praised the efficacy of the calcium scan or lamented that too few are covered by insurance: "If the press picks up on this topic and makes heart scanning a household word, millions of unnecessary premature deaths could be avoided." A few were not enthusiastic: "The coronary calcium score is hype. . . . there isn't any good data on how calcium scores correlate to prognosis." Most also believed strongly in statins (though, again, a few didn't). One doctor, clearly in the statin camp, declared that going forward, people like me with my heart history should be put on them preventively, at age twenty.

One woman sent me her recipe for oat-bran muffins. A man sent me a picture of himself with his eleven-year-old daughter at the 85-mile mark of a 135-mile charity bicycle ride. For inspiration someone passed along a short bio of Fred Lebow, the "Mad Genius" behind the New York City Marathon. Another person, noting my 6-foot-8-inch height, asked me about graduation rates on college basketball teams.

Six people wrote extolling the benefits of chelation therapy, a treatment for removing heavy metals from the bloodstream. "Your experience with orthodox medicine and their approach is what one would expect. Allopathic medicine uses the 'poison, slash, and burn' approach for all their patients. Not good!" Chelation, these e-mails said, also is useful in stripping plaque from arteries. Another e-mailer, however, wrote to say his father had turned to chelation. His cholesterol did go down, but the son attributed this to the fact that his dad previously had also radically changed his diet. In any event, he said, the doctor treating his father with chelation had refused to order an autopsy. "Not a good sign," the son wrote.

I was told to take Omega-3, salmon oil, Coenzyme Q-10 and flaxseed oil, as well as vitamins B-6 and B-12. I was told also to take massive doses of folic acid; and blueberries, cherries, and acai (a Brazilian fruit) in pill form. To restrict my caloric intake, two people recommended alternate-day fasting. It was recommended that I eat Alaskan wild salmon three times a week, drink a glass of pomegranate juice a day, and eat organic kale and onions for their antioxidant value. And red yeast rice; more than a few people recommended red yeast rice, a statin in natural form.

There was even the occasional Bible verse, often sent with no further explanation: 1 Kings 3:14—*"And if you walk in my ways and obey my statutes and commands as David your father did, I will give you a long life."* (New International Version)

I was grateful for every e-mail. For the fact alone that people took the time to write. For the hugely important lesson these many missives, together and separately, imparted. I learned that I wasn't alone. That I am no expert. That people feel as strongly about their way of living a healthy life as they do about their children or their pets. I mean no disrespect; I am not being flip. I learned that if I wanted to write a book—and I also learned that I needed to write a book—the only story I could tell, had the right to tell, was my own, Dad's own, our family's own.

I was warned that a stress test doesn't provide much information if the blockage in an artery is below about 70 percent. I was reminded that there can be false positives in the calcium scores. It was suggested that I next do an echocardiogram; a nuclear-imaging stress test; a VAP cholesterol test (a "vertical auto profile"; it breaks out the LDL and HDL into further subtypes). One doctor said I needed to get an angiogram "as soon as you can"; another ordered a heart bypass operation "NOW!"

A few wrote with the hint that I lacked the courage to go it alone without a statin. They are right. Though not that I didn't consider it, at least in theory. I even toyed with this silly thought: since they weren't available to Dad, then I shouldn't avail myself of them now. Taking a drug would be letting him down, breaking my promise. I did think that. I am not a grassy-knoll conspiracy type, but I was also tempted to work up a fever over the pharmaceutical companies and the money they make and the cahooting they do, or at least what the rumors say they do.

In the real world I had to realize I had no good alternative. Not with my family history. My father; my grandfather; my great-grandfather and his "apoplexy." And my great-great-grandfather, too, a John McKee born in Ireland who came to Philadelphia in 1850. He died in 1896 of "valvular heart disease," says the coroner's certificate. He was sixty-six years old—to date in America the longest-lived McKee male in my direct line. There were Dad's three McKee uncles, who with fourth brother Jack all died in a twelve-year span beginning in 1941. This quartet of heart attacks speaks loudly to me, at near the decibel level of Dad's own. And there were Dad's two sisters, Mary Jane and Alice, who both died peacefully in their sleep. Exploring further branches of the McKee tree and it becomes almost comical. A cousin once removed died before age forty; a great aunt in her early thirties. On and on. Stop it, you're killing me.

Everything else being equal, if there was something else I could have done before doing a drug I would have done it. But I don't smoke, so I couldn't make the grandest gesture of all by quitting. I could lose five or six pounds, bringing my body-mass index down a couple, three points, but it wasn't like there was room for a makeover. I could always eat better. Everyone can always eat better. But as one e-mailer wrote: "My doctor . . . said, 'With your family history you can eat cardboard all day and still have high cholesterol.'" As for those twenty-five years of working out, I already was in great shape. But maybe I could get in better shape. Yes, that was it! I could study up for another stress test, blow past John Carlos and Peter Norman into Tommie Smith gold-medal territory. I thought that, too. Sure I did. But no. Another thousand meters on the rowing machine wasn't going to make the difference.

So I went on a statin.

Inside of a week I felt like I'd been beaten with a baseball bat. I'd be sitting at my desk at work and I'd stand up and for a second, just half a second, really, this great wave of satisfaction would roll through me because my body felt as if that morning I had put myself through the single hardest workout of my entire life. Everything about me ached. I must have really nailed it at the gym! There is no feeling quite like it, there really isn't.

Except, no, that wasn't it. I had heart disease, and I was on some drug because I couldn't go it alone anymore. And now I could barely walk because of it, barely keep my hands up at the keyboard, barely bend over at the water cooler. And that great wave of satisfaction would crash upon me and pummel me under its dread. This was my life, after all I had done? I called the doctor. He told me to come in for a blood test the next morning. I did, and that afternoon he called to tell me to get off the drug *immediately*. He said come back in a month and we'd try something else, at the lowest dose. Within another month my cholesterol had fallen through the floor, HDLs and LDLs in the right place. Best of all, no side effects that I could tell.

This was, however, in its own way the final indignity. I can say I almost wish the drug hadn't worked. Ego and arrogance talking. A sports analogy to try to explain. I understand Ray Bourque now. The hockey player spent nearly twenty-one seasons with the Boston Bruins—indeed, he came to BE the Boston Bruins. But through all those years of glory and struggle he never won the Stanley Cup; he came close twice, but he never did. So at age thirty-nine he asked the Bruins for a trade and they obliged, to the Colorado Avalanche, and the next year he won his Stanley Cup. Every player on the championship team gets one day to do with the Cup whatever he wants. On his day, Ray Bourque took it back to Boston, to celebrate with 15,000 Bruins fans at City Hall Plaza. He'd finally won the Cup and good for him. It just wasn't the way he'd always thought it would be.

My angsting out over statins in the *Journal* article precipitated its own round of e-mails. A few commiserated. "My initial reaction was anger and resistance. I felt betrayed," wrote one. Said another: "I fought taking medication, too, believing it represented a failure to do enough myself." A few more scolded me, telling me to get over myself, shut up and take the drug. "We're very lucky to be living in a time of great medical breakthroughs," I was reminded by one. Another was more direct: "Smile Steve, take your meds." Admonished a third: "I think you're too hard on yourself—you can fight your own gene pool only so much. You do the best you can, and if you can get some aid from modern medicine, do it, and do it with gratitude."

But of the 226 e-mails I received, fully 111 of them began with words like these:

> *I could have written that essay. . . . If you changed the names, it would be my story. . . . I, too, am my father's son. . . . I am my father's daughter. . . . There are so many parallels between your story and mine it is scary. . . . I too am a cardiac legacy. . . . I could have been reading about myself. . . . I read it as a history of my own family. . . .*

And on and on. There was the man whose father died while putting toys together for his nine children on Christmas Eve. Another man spoke of being, at forty-six, "the old man of the family." His father died at thirty-eight; his grandfather at forty; his brother at thirty-six. "I sit at the head of the table," he wrote. "I carve the turkey." One woman wrote to say, "My mother died at the age of 50 of a sudden heart attack when I was 17. My brother died at the age of 40 and my father at 68. Another brother has had bypass surgery."

One man's father died in 1960 at age forty-six. "I was 18," he said. Now he does everything he can, but he is sixty-three "and

[I] often ask myself how I can be so old." This was a common theme. We "cardiac legacies," we know the math by heart. "I am 60 now," wrote one, "having outlived my father by 14 years, or 30% percent longer than he lived." Another said: "I'm now 58, and for the past 9 years I have felt like I was on borrowed time." And there was this: "I'm 71 now, and was just 16 when my father died in 1950 at the age of 53. . . . I'm sure, as most people I suspect are when they lose a parent of the same sex very early on, that I would suffer the same fate." Yes, we do. "I am 20 years your junior," wrote one e-mailer. "My father had his first blowout at 49. . . . It is not ironic that his episode occurred at the same age of his father's first attack. I have come to think of 49 as my scarlet number!"

But mostly in these e-mails there was hope.

"I am now 58," wrote a man whose father had died at forty seven, ". . . and I am now enjoying my first grandchild." Wrote a man whose father had died at fifty: "My cholesterol is <150 and I aim to keep it there. I work out every day. I sweat out my fear on the treadmill, trying to keep ahead of what I hope will not be my fate as well." Another man came at it all from a very unexpected direction, after "battling my genes since I was 19." He was doing all he could, but there was still more to do. "I have been trying to defy it by reading all I can about all of the countries in the world, the classics in literature, art and music. It has become a compulsion for me to learn as much as I can about life. I had become a coward but am now starting to take some chances. . . . I hope sometime to have the chance to see, in person, some of the beautiful works of art I have been reading about. . . . I still sometime live in fear, but I am trying to look into its face without turning away."

Finally, there was this from a man who was twenty years old when his father died at age fifty. His dad's name was John Mc-Kee. "It is amazing how many similarities we have," he wrote. "I truly hope that we share at least one more: that we both break the short life cycle of McKee men and live long lives so we can share the memories of our fathers with our kids so they are not forgotten."

That's all this was, this book, an attempt to share the memory of my father.

I have since that first calcium test had two annual follow-ups. When the first-year's follow-up came in thirty points under that 452, my doctor was pleased but cautious. One or the other could be a statistical anomaly. It was the second year, when my number came in again at 452, that he expressed delight. It was likely now that I wasn't producing any new plaque, any vulnerable plaque, he said. It was tempting then to ask him if I could go off the statin, but I already knew his answer.

To use Dr. Fein's word, I was "thrilled" with this second follow-up, this second 452. I was on a drug, yes, but I had also for the past two years kept up the exercise, ramped it up, actually. I had started taking niacin, a B-vitamin, as a second cholesterol reducer. I was on a daily aspirin. I had stayed with the psyllium cereal and the plant-stanol spread. I had added a fiber supplement (more psyllium), Omega-3s, flaxseed, Coenzyme Q-10, and more fish to the diet. I've recently had an echocardiogram as well, this on the advice of my family doctor. In a final piece of irony, writing *My Father's Heart*—living with it for more than a year—raised my blood pressure. At least that's how I diagnosed it. The echo indicated a slight thickening of my left ventricle—the power chamber (though the doctor conceded my 6-feet-8-inches might itself be the reason). This raised the specter of another decision on another drug. But for now my answer was no, not more. Besides, a checkup with the doctor two weeks after I pushed the button on all nine chapters, clearing them from my desk, and my blood pressure was perfectly normal. This is a journey after all; never ending.

In the meantime, there was a triathlon to finish. This was a "reverse" tri—it started with the run, went to the bike, and ended with the swim. Some experienced triathlon friends frowned on this sequence. With good reason. The swim should be first, they said, so that no one is too tired in the water, so no one . . . drowns. Nothing like that happened here. But the pool was a giant "L" shape, the bottom falling away at the far end, and the first time I swam over it I got disoriented by the sudden deep. The rest of my eight laps I concentrated literally on the very next stroke of my arm, picturing my hand coming out of the water behind me, over the top, then back in the pool. Every movement purposeful, time itself meaningless, no past, no future, just the placement of my fingers right now. Like with the Equinox twenty-four years before, the goal was to finish, and I did.

Everything about this triathlon took me wonderfully by surprise. While in training, I felt completely rejuvenated, calling on all the fitness I had banked through all those years. It had been worth it after all. How could I have doubted it? I hired a friend who does tri training as a hobby, put myself totally in his hands, did whatever he told me. Having someone else to blame when doing Dad's road work was ridiculously freeing.

But what surprised me most was what awaited me when Noreen and I arrived at Patrick's school. I had promised myself that once I got to the race, I would low-key it. Be the grownup here, make this about Patrick and his first race. Except the night before he told me he planned to run the five-kilometer first leg with me. "Dad," he said, "I know you're a really slow runner." Making *this* the most left-handed compliment I have ever heard. His plan, he said, was to do the run with me. That way he wouldn't get himself out too fast, ahead of himself, and have to pay the price later. I tried to dissuade him, however half-heartedly, but he insisted. To be in the same race with him was going to be terrific enough. But to run with him?

Patrick is diabetic. When he came to us I remember thinking that because he was adopted the McKee genes wouldn't be visited upon him. I thought this in so many words and was glad for it. I was correct, too. What I didn't know until he taught me a few years ago is that we are who we are, whoever that is.

So now here he was at the beginning of this race, still running backward, still spinning his hands, still grinning. I caught up to him, he turned around, and we settled in. As Patrick had predicted, my pace had put us near the end of the pack, just the two of us. Father and son, shoulder to shoulder, out for a run. *You're still here, Steve, you're still here.* The only sound was the *crunch-crunch-crunch* of the gravel beneath our feet.

ACKNOWLEDGMENTS

I would first like to thank the people who appear in these pages who talked with me about the old days of the York Crowd, camping, hunting and fishing, Haines Acres, St. Joe's, Buffalo, and all the rest. Everyone gave generously of their time. I am extremely grateful to each of you.

Marnie Cochran, my editor at Da Capo Press, always understood what kind of book this needed to become. Her care, guidance, and encouragement were critical as she waited almost a year for me to get it there. Renee Sedliar at Da Capo has been a terrific editor and sounding board as this project rounded into form through its final stages. I am very grateful to both of them for their enthusiasm and commitment to *My Father's Heart*.

I would also like to thank Renee Caputo, the project editor, for her diligent work transforming the manuscript into an actual book. And from one copy editor to another, I would like to thank Martin Hanft for his meticulous and much-appreciated performance.

My agent, Jeff Kleinman, at Folio Literary Management has been from the get-go a relentlessly hard worker in behalf of this book. He's amazing. *My Father's Heart* would not have come to life without him. Thanks, Jeff. I need also to thank Steve Sax, the former Los Angeles Dodger, and Ken Wells, a former editor at the *Wall Street Journal*, for helping to put in place the circumstances by which Jeff and I came to work together.

At the *Wall Street Journal* I must first thank senior editor Larry Rout, the editor of the *Journal Report*. His venue provided the foundation for *My Father's Heart*; his guidance proved invaluable. John Blanton, Bart Zeigler, and Don Arbour served at various times as the editors for the two articles that appeared in these reports. Christine Glancey was at the beginning of this project the *Journal*'s global copy chief. Her immediate and complete enthusiasm when I asked for the time off to write this book will always mean a great deal to me. Assistant Managing Editor Al Anspaugh also needed to sign off on my leave of absence, and he did so with great encouragement. And I should thank Michael Boone, Christine's successor on the copy desk, for waiting patiently (I believe) when my leave extended beyond my original request. Paul Steiger, the managing editor when I started this project, created the atmosphere that allows *Journal* people to pursue such dreams as this. Marcus Brauchli, the managing editor when I returned, has sustained it. Finally, at the *Journal* I would like to thank Jim Pensiero and colleague and friend Stefan Fatsis. And Jim McDonald and Christian Talag of the Dow Jones Help Desk, who provided invaluable IT support.

James McClure, the editor of the *York Daily Record* and a Pennsylvania historian, provided great encouragement and many terrific ideas and suggestions when this project was in its earliest stages. He also read closely the York Crowd sections of the book.

Nicole Ouellet spent her 2007 "winter term" for Oberlin College as my personal researcher, running down every question I could think to ask her. She wasn't just interested, she was curious. Thank you, Nic.

I spent two weeks total at the York County Heritage Trust Historical Society Museum and Library Archives, at the Buffalo and Erie County Historical Society, and at the Lackawanna Historical Society in Scranton. Josh Stahlman in York, Patricia M. Virgil in Buffalo, and Bob Booth in Scranton were immensely helpful . . . and patient. I would like also to thank Richard Stanislaus of the Pennsylvania Anthracite Heritage Museum in Scranton.

Jane McGinley, Carey Steward, and Jim McKee graciously granted access to the findings of their thoroughly researched McKee family tree. In similar fashion, information from a comprehensive Brady/O'Neil family tree was provided courtesy P. Barry Cotter, M.D., Mary Anne Gannon, Thomas H. Healy, and Jo Ann Tuskin. The generosity of these people spared me untold hours of work, and I am grateful to all of them.

Thanks go to McKee cousins Joanne Murphy Beringer and all the Gampps—Edwin, Ann LaPorta, Mary, Eileen Lew, and Susanne. Also, Myra O'Malley Howley. And O'Neil cousins Ann Callaghan Zorn, Jennifer Zorn Cox and her husband, Brian, and Tom O'Brien.

Vicky Vossen and Pat Hansen provided a close and considered reading of the manuscript. Tim Carroll of the *Wall Street*

Journal Global Copy Desk and Toula Polygalaktos brought their professional eye to bear on a careful reading of the book in galley form.

Therese Warden in Buffalo and Terri Eline in York did much-appreciated legwork. Therese's son, the Rev. Fr. Joel M. Warden, C.O., translated The Lord's Prayer into Greek; Terri, an English teacher at York Catholic High School, also read the manuscript.

At York Hospital in Pennsylvania, W. Jay Nicholson, M.D., Keith Noll, Barry Sparks, and Laura Place were very generous with their time and resources.

Many thanks to the staff of the Princeton Longevity Center, including Bernadette Sushko, Christopher J. Volgraf, Karen McPartland, and Andrea Lanza.

I contacted a quartet of former employees at Cole Steel, who spoke with me under an agreement of anonymity. I would like to thank them for bringing that place alive for me again, providing the details of Otto Lewin's life, and walking me through Dad's day in the warehouse.

In like manner, the men and women who described their heart-attack experiences and the doctors and hospital administrator who "diagnosed" Dad's fatal attack also spoke knowing that they would receive no formal credit for their time and insights. I am grateful to all of them.

All errors are my own. I reviewed many research details with a number of people, including: Dan Dilandro, college archivist at Buffalo State College. Phyllis Camesano, public relations director, Buffalo State. Patricia Donovan, senior editor, Office of

News Services, University at Buffalo. Mike Strong in York, who read the Civil War, Baltimore Colts, and York sections. Martha Shulski of the Alaska Climate Research Center and Amy Hartley, information officer of the Geophysical Institute at the University of Alaska–Fairbanks. Christina Novak, director of communications, Pennsylvania Department of Conservation and Natural Resources. John H. Kaercher, environmental education specialist, Little Pine State Park, Waterville, Pennsylvania. Karen Rayer, International Bible Society. Deborah Pettibone, office of public affairs at the Roswell Park Cancer Institute, Buffalo. Gayle Houck, grants office manager, the John R. Oishei Foundation. John Estle and the extremely comprehensive Fairbanks Equinox Marathon website www.equinoxmarathon.org provided a wealth of race details.

In addition I would like to acknowledge: Conrad Kiffin. Julie Downey. Anne Downey. Alice Beal. Edna Pytlak. Bob Schlehr. The Keffer Funeral Home. Donald Epstein. Sister Marian Dolores Franz, I.H.M. Sister St. Michel Mullany, I.H.M. Rev. Edward J. Sheedy, Christ the King Seminary, Buffalo. George Trout. Richard Collier. Matthew Fenwick, American Hospital Association. B. J. Spigelmyer, sports information director at DeSales University, and Scott Coval, the men's basketball coach. Scott Frey, the sports information director at Messiah College. Natasha Bedingfield, Danielle Brisebois, and Wayne Rodrigues. Joe Miceli, a York Catholic classmate who stopped by the house on Wednesday night when I was at Gino's with Mary Liz. Carol Jacoby at WGAL-TV Channel 8, Lancaster, Pennsylvania. Jim Horn at WSBA radio in York.

Cheryl Hofsummer, Cathedral Cemetery, Scranton. Fran Keller, Martin Memorial Library in York.

Finally, to Noreen and Patrick: Thanks for everything, absolutely everything.

AN UPDATE

Allentown College of St. Francis de Sales was renamed DeSales University on January 1, 2001. The mascot changed from the Centaur to the Bulldog. The school remains located in Center Valley, Pennsylvania.

A NOTE ON THE NUMBERS

Data regarding cardiovascular disease, coronary heart disease, and sudden cardiac arrest in the United States provided by the American Heart Association's (AHA) "Heart Disease and Stroke Statistics—2007 Update." The report's findings are a compilation of research from the Centers for Disease Control and Prevention's (CDC) National Center for Health Statistics (NCHS); the National Institutes of Health's National Heart, Lung, and Blood Institute (NHLBI); the National Institute of Neurological Disorders and Stroke; and other government agencies. Further statistics provided by the studies "Men and Heart Disease" and "Women and Heart Disease," cooperative reports by the CDC and the Office for Social Environment and Health Research, West Virginia University in Morgantown. Data on ambulance calls during heart attacks from the AHA.

Statistics on smoking and tobacco provided by the AHA, the NCHS, the Department of Health and Human Service's "2005 National Survey on Drug Use and Health," and NHLBI's "Morbidity & Mortality: 2004 Chart Book on Cardiovascular, Lung and Blood Diseases." Historical data on smoking prevalence in 1949 and 1969 from the Gallup Organization.

320